Food Facts for Older Adults

Introduction

AF754536

What should you eat to stay healthy? New information about nutrition seems to come out each day. Often, the information does not address the concerns of older adults. Sometimes the advice is confusing. This bulletin focuses on nutrition topics of particular interest to older adults and gives suggestions on how you can improve your diet by following the Dietary Guidelines for Americans.

The Dietary Guidelines for Americans

- Eat a variety of foods
- Maintain healthy weight
- Choose a diet low in fat, saturated fat, and cholesterol
- Choose a diet with plenty of vegetables, fruits, and grain products
- Use sugars only in moderation
- Use salt and sodium only in moderation
- If you drink alcoholic beverages, do so in moderation

Sorting out information on nutrition, figuring out what it means for you personally, and making changes in how you eat are well worth the effort. What you eat may affect your risk for several of the leading causes of death in the United States, such as coronary heart disease, stroke, diabetes, and some types of cancer. More importantly, healthy eating and regular exercise can give you the energy and strength to enjoy an active, independent lifestyle as long as possible.

Americans of all ages need to eat healthier. Making changes doesn't have to be difficult. You don't have to give up your favorite foods or stop eating out. With some basic information and a look at your current eating habits, you can begin to make gradual changes that can help you improve or maintain your health.

This bulletin provides information and suggestions that can help you follow the guidelines, including—

1. facts about fat, cholesterol, and sodium;

2. a discussion of the special needs of older adults, including getting enough nutrients, fluids, and fiber, and precautions when taking medications;

3. tips on making healthy food choices when you shop and cook;

4. how to maintain a healthy weight;

5. questions older people ask about nutrition;

6. a roundup of tips and recipes for preparing foods Dietary Guidelines style; and

7. a list of resources for more information.

Please note that this information is for people who are generally in good health. If your doctor has prescribed a special diet for you because of a health conditon, follow that advice. However, this bulletin will help you better understand current nutrition information and may raise questions for you to discuss with your doctor or dietitian about your special nutrition needs.

Food Facts for Older Adults

What You Should Know About Fat, Cholesterol, and Sodium

1

Every day you hear some news items about fat, cholesterol, or sodium. What should you know about them, and what should you do about them when making food choices?

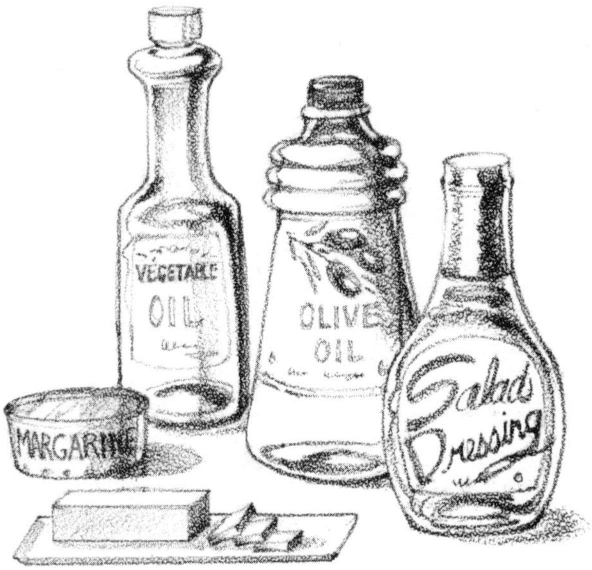

Some Facts About Fat and Cholesterol

Fats are the most concentrated source of food energy (calories). Fats are mixtures of three kinds of fatty acids—saturated, monounsaturated, and polyunsaturated. A fat that contains a lot of saturated fatty acids is usually firm, like butter or lard. Some vegetable fats like coconut oil, palm kernel oil, and palm oil are also high in saturated fatty acids. Vegetable oils such as olive oil, canola oil, corn oil, or soybean oil contain a lot of monounsaturated and polyunsaturated fatty acids. When vegetable oils are hydrogenated to form solid shortenings or margarine, some of the unsaturated fatty acids become saturated, and the fat becomes firm.

> ***DID YOU KNOW???***
>
> Some fat is necessary in the diet. It provides energy, helps your body absorb vitamins such as A, D, and E, and provides essential fatty acids needed by everyone in small amounts. Fat also helps make food taste good, providing flavor, aroma, and texture.

Cholesterol is a fatlike substance found in almost all your body cells. Your body can make it, but it also comes from the food you eat. Cholesterol is present in all animal foods—meat, poultry, fish, dairy products, and egg yolks. Both the cholesterol that comes from your food (dietary cholesterol) and the cholesterol made by your body circulate in your blood (blood cholesterol). Cholesterol is used by your body to make hormones, substances needed for digestion, and new cells.

Try A Stirfry

Stirfrying is a quick and easy cooking method that requires very little fat. Heat a heavy skillet or a wok and add just enough oil to lightly coat the bottom of the pan—about 1 or 2 teaspoons. Then add the food and stir constantly while cooking. Start with thin strips or diced portions of meat, poultry, or fish. When the meat is almost done, add small pieces of vegetables such as broccoli, cauliflower, zucchini, sprouts, carrots, mushrooms, tomatoes, or green onions. Cook just until vegetables are tender, but still crisp and bright in color. For a slightly softer texture, add about 2 tablespoons of water, cover the pan, and steam for a few minutes.

Why Be Concerned About Fat and Cholesterol?

If you have a high blood cholesterol level, you have a greater chance of having a heart attack or a stroke. Eating too much saturated fat, cholesterol, and too many calories can increase your blood cholesterol. A diet containing too much **total** fat and too many calories may increase your risk for certain cancers.

The way diet affects blood cholesterol varies among individuals. However, blood cholesterol does increase in most people when they eat a diet high in saturated fat and cholesterol and excessive in calories. Of these, dietary saturated fat has the greatest effect; dietary cholesterol has less.

Should You Be Concerned?

A blood cholesterol level of 200 mg/dl or less is considered desirable for adults. The relation of blood cholesterol to the risk for heart disease is less clear in older adults than in middle-aged people. However, heart disease is still the number one cause of death in older Americans, both men and women. Smoking, high blood pressure, diabetes, lack of exercise, heredity, and being overweight are other risk factors. If you don't know what your blood cholesterol level is, ask your doctor to check it the next time you go for a visit. Your doctor can help you evaluate your risk and determine whether your cholesterol level is too high. Your doctor can also explain the different kinds of blood cholesterol (HDL and LDL), triglycerides, and other blood lipids and explain how they affect your risk for heart disease.

Most of us eat too much fat. Even if your blood cholesterol level is not high, you may want to make some changes in your food choices to reduce the amount of fat and saturated fat you eat. If you're like most Americans, 36 percent of your calories come from fat. A diet with 30 percent or less of calories from total fat (**and** less than 10 percent of calories from saturated fat) would be healthier. Reducing fat may help you control your weight if necessary. This is important because obesity increases your risk for high blood pressure, stroke, high blood cholesterol, and diabetes and also aggravates arthritis by putting added stress on your joints.

DID YOU KNOW???

Fat is not the same as cholesterol. Some foods contain a lot of cholesterol, but are low in fat, like liver; and some foods have no cholesterol, but are high in fat, like nondairy creamers, vegetable oil, or margarine. A food that says "no cholesterol" can still be high in fat. Read the label to see how much and which kinds of fats are included in the product before you buy it.

All types of fat have the same number of calories—both butter and margarine have about 36 calories per teaspoon. So, go easy on all fats and foods made with a lot of fat.

Easy Ways To Cut Fat, Saturated Fat, and Cholesterol in Your Diet

At the Store:

- Choose lean cuts of meat, such as beef round, loin, sirloin, pork loin chops, and roasts.
- Consider fish and poultry as alternatives; they are somewhat lower in saturated fat.
- Buy lowfat versions of dairy products.
- Read the food label and choose those foods that are lower in fat, saturated fat, and cholesterol.

At the Table:

- Use less of **all** fats and oils, especially saturated fats such as butter, cream, sour cream, and cream cheese.
- Try reduced-calorie salad dressings—they are usually low in fat.
- As a beverage, gradually replace whole milk with 2 percent fat milk, then 1 percent fat or skim milk.

In the Kitchen:

- When cooking, replace saturated fats such as butter and lard with small amounts of polyunsaturated and monounsaturated fats in vegetable oils such as corn oil, soybean oil, olive oil, peanut oil, or canola oil.
- Broil, roast, bake, steam, or boil foods instead of frying them, or try stirfrying (see box on page 4) with just a little fat.
- Trim all visible fat from meats before cooking and remove the skin from poultry.
- Spoon off fat from meat dishes after they are cooked.
- Use skim milk or lowfat milk when making "cream" sauces, soups, or puddings.
- Substitute lowfat yogurt or whipped lowfat cottage cheese for sour cream and mayonnaise in dips and dressings.
- Substitute two egg whites for each whole egg in recipes for most quick breads, cookies, and cakes. (The cholesterol and fat are in the yolk, not in the white.)
- Try lemon juice, herbs, or spices to season foods instead of butter or margarine.

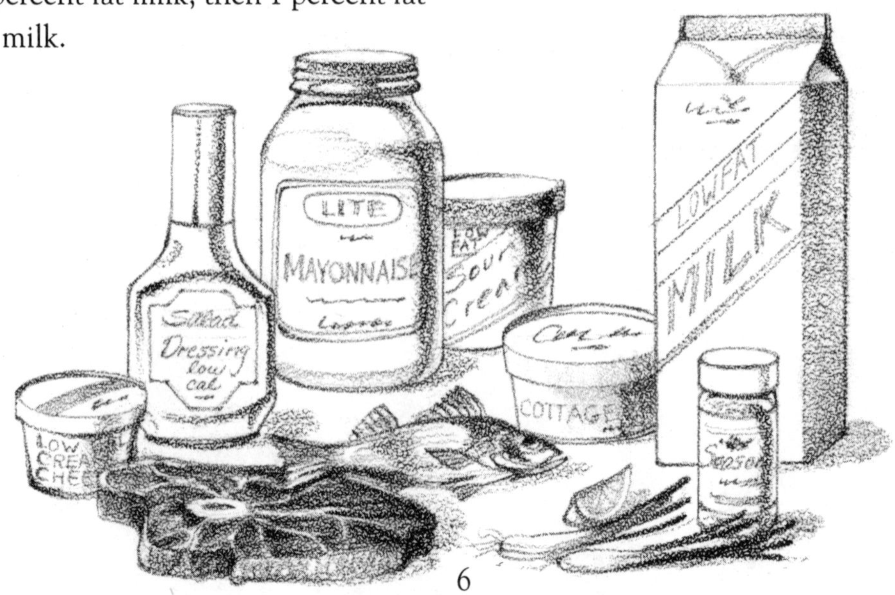

Some Facts About Sodium

Sodium occurs naturally in most foods. It is also added to many foods and beverages, usually as salt. One teaspoon of salt contains about 2,000 milligrams of sodium. The body needs sodium to maintain normal blood volume and for the nerves and muscles. But, populations with diets high in salt have more high blood pressure, a condition that increases your risk for heart attack, stroke, and kidney disease. People with high blood pressure are usually advised to restrict their salt and sodium. It is also important to maintain a healthy weight, exercise regularly, and stay on your medication.

No one can predict who will develop high blood pressure, but many Americans eat more sodium than they actually need. Some health authorities suggest that healthy adults try to limit their sodium intake to 2,400 milligrams (mg) a day.

Much of the sodium in the American diet comes from salt added in cooking or at the table. The taste for salt is learned—you can "unlearn" it by gradually cutting down on your salt intake. Start by thinking about how much sodium you add every time you use that salt shaker.

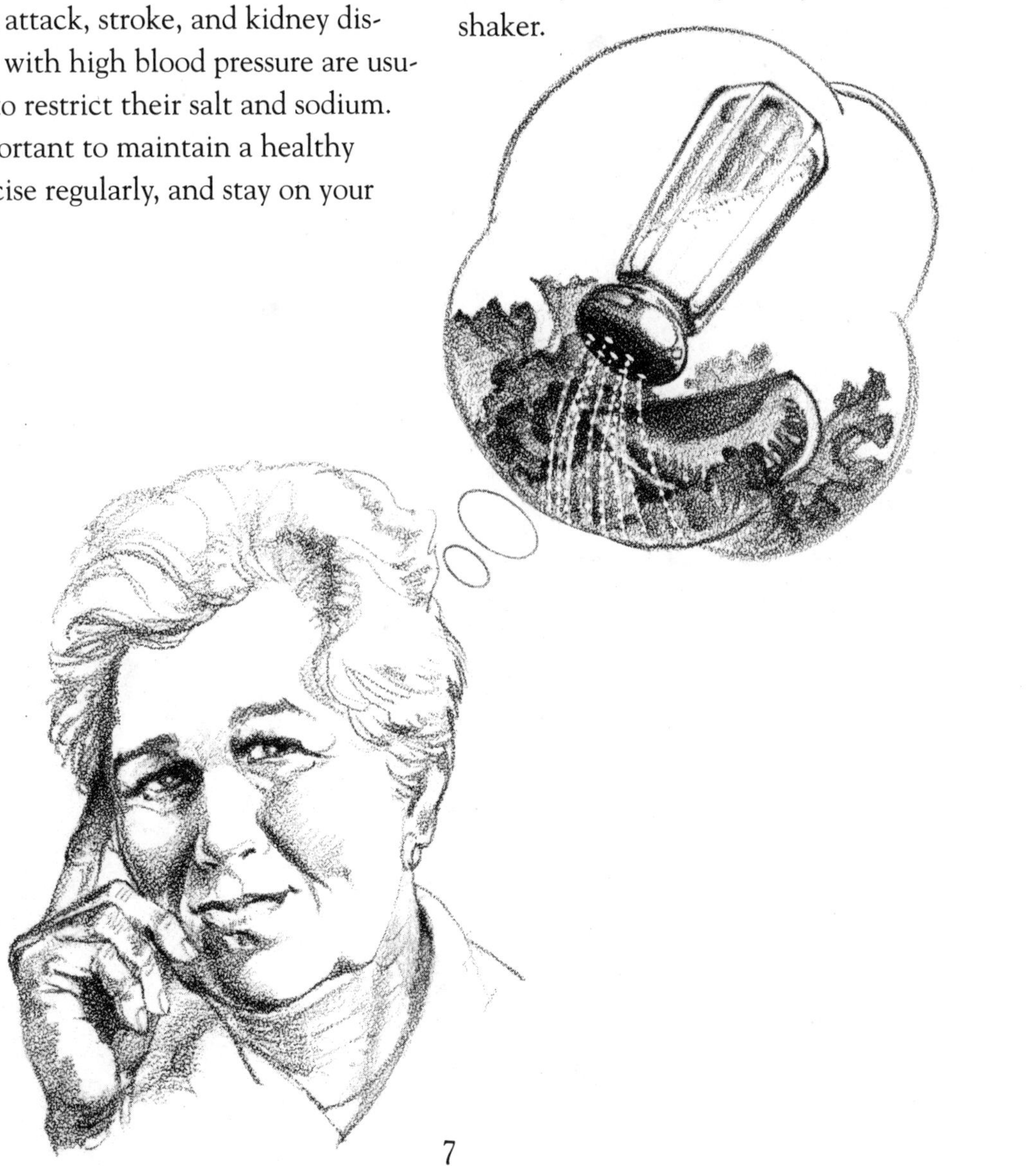

Sodium is an ingredient in many foods—even ones that might not taste salty, such as luncheon meats, ready-to-eat cereals, and many mixes and prepared foods at the supermarket. Sodium is found in soy sauce and other prepared sauces and dressings, cured meats, canned soups and vegetables, most cheeses, and many convenience foods such as frozen dinners and casserole mixes.

> ***DID YOU KNOW???***
>
> Salt substitutes are not for everyone. People who are under medical supervision, particularly for kidney problems, should check with their doctor before using salt substitutes.
>
> Try commercial seasoning blends that are mixtures of spices and herbs without added salt. These, as well as homemade seasoning blends, can be used to flavor foods without adding sodium.

Some Tips on Reducing Sodium in Your Diet:

At the Store:

- Read labels for information on the sodium content (see Section 3 for more information on food labels).
- Try fresh or plain frozen vegetables and meats instead of those canned or prepared with salt.
- Look for low or reduced sodium or "no-salt-added" versions of foods.

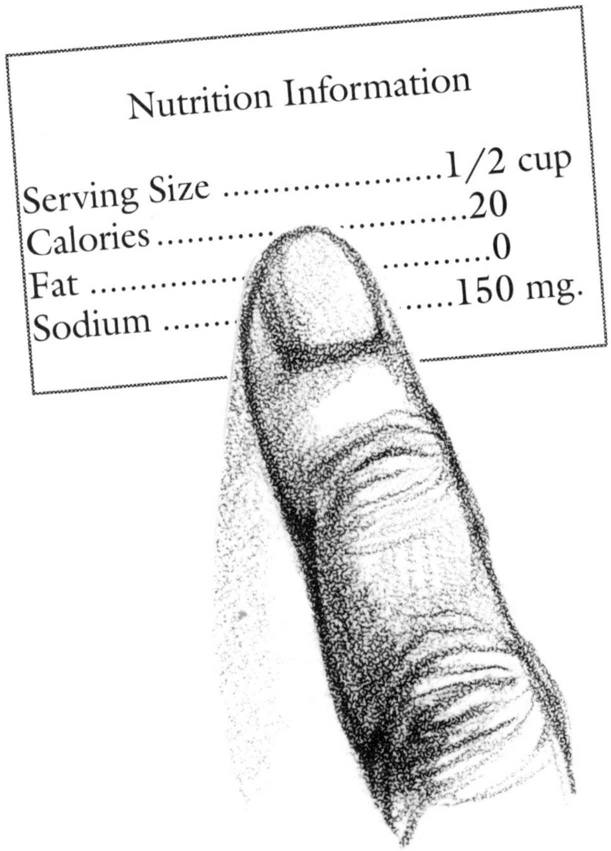

In the Kitchen:

- Cook plain rice, pasta, and hot cereals using less salt than the package calls for (try 1/8 teaspoon of salt for two servings). "Instant" rice, pasta, and cereals may contain salt added by the processor.
- Adjust your recipes, gradually cutting down on the amount of salt. If some of the ingredients already contain salt, such as canned soup or vegetables, you may not need to add any more salt at all.
- Use herbs and spices as seasonings for vegetables and meats instead of salt.

At the Table:

- Taste your food before you salt it. Does it really need more salt? Try one shake instead of two. Gradually cut down on the amount of salt you use. Your taste will adjust to less salt.

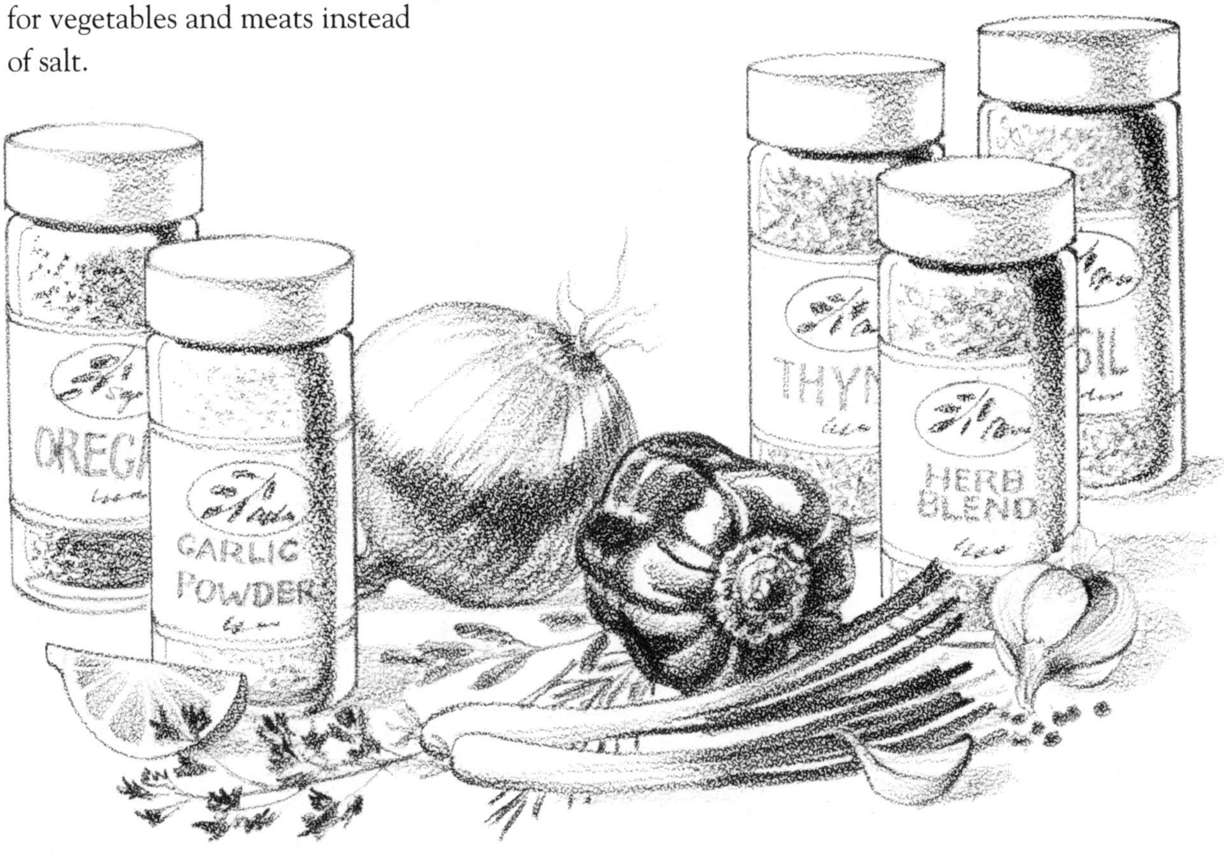

Where's the Salt?

The following table will give you an idea of the amount of sodium in different types of food. Individual products vary. Information on food labels can also help you make choices to moderate your sodium intake.

WHERE'S THE SALT?

FOOD GROUP	SODIUM, milligrams
BREADS, CEREALS	
Cooked cereal, rice, pasta, unsalted	trace per 1/2 cup
Ready-to-eat cereal	100-350 per oz.
Bread	110-175 per slice
FRUITS	
Fruit, fresh, frozen, canned	trace per 1/2 cup
VEGETABLES	
Vegetables, fresh or frozen cooked without salt	less than 70 per 1/2 cup
Vegetables, canned, or frozen with sauce	140-460 per 1/2 cup
Tomato juice, canned	660 per 3/4 cup
Vegetable soup, canned	810 per cup
MEAT, POULTRY, FISH	
Fresh meat, poultry, fish	less than 90 per 3 oz.
Tuna, canned, water pack	300 per 3 oz.
Bologna	580 per 2 oz.
Ham, lean roasted	1,025 per 3 oz.
MILK, YOGURT, CHEESE	
Milk	120 per cup
Yogurt	170 per 8 oz.
Natural cheeses, such as Cheddar or swiss	110-275 per 1-1/2 oz.
Process cheeses, such as American or swiss	790 per 2 oz.
OTHER	
Salad dressing	80-220 per tbsp.
Catsup, steak sauce	180-230 per tbsp.
Soy sauce	1,020 per tbsp.
Salt	2,000 per tsp.
Dill pickle	930 per 1 medium
Potato chips, salted	135 per oz.
Corn chips, salted	235 per oz.
Peanuts, roasted in oil, salted	120 per oz.

Summing Up:

It's natural to think about fat, saturated fat, cholesterol, or sodium as separate parts of your diet, but the best idea is to look at your diet as a whole. You can have small amounts of any food as part of a balanced diet. For example, if one of your food choices is relatively high in fat and sodium, such as baked ham, choose low fat and low sodium foods to eat with it, such as fresh or plain frozen vegetables cooked with little salt and seasoned with herbs instead of butter or margarine.

A Food Choice Checkup

Think about your own food choices. Use these quizzes to check your diet for fat and sodium and see where you might begin to make some small changes as suggested in this section.

How do you score on FAT?

How often do you eat—	Seldom or never	1 to 2 times a week	3 to 5 times a week	Almost daily
1. Fried, deep-fat fried, or breaded foods?	☐	☐	☐	☐
2. Fatty meats, such as sausage, luncheon meats, fatty steaks and roasts?	☐	☐	☐	☐
3. Whole milk, high-fat cheeses, ice cream?	☐	☐	☐	☐
4. Pies, pastries, rich cakes?	☐	☐	☐	☐
5. Rich cream sauces and gravies?	☐	☐	☐	☐
6. Oily salad dressings, mayonnaise?	☐	☐	☐	☐
7. Butter or margarine on vegetables, dinner rolls, toast?	☐	☐	☐	☐

How do you score on SODIUM?

How often do you—	Seldom or never	1 to 2 times a week	3 to 5 times a week	Almost daily
1. Eat cured or processed meats, such as ham, sausage, frankfurters, and other luncheon meats?	☐	☐	☐	☐
2. Choose canned vegetables or frozen vegetables with sauce?	☐	☐	☐	☐
3. Use frozen TV dinners, entrees, or canned or dehydrated soups?	☐	☐	☐	☐
4. Eat cheese?	☐	☐	☐	☐
5. Eat salted nuts, popcorn, pretzels, corn chips, or potato chips?	☐	☐	☐	☐
6. Add salt to cooking water for vegetables, rice, pasta, or cereals, or add seasoning mixes or sauces containing salt when preparing foods?	☐	☐	☐	☐
7. Salt your food before tasting it?	☐	☐	☐	☐

Take a look at your answers.

Several checks in the last two columns mean you may have a high fat or sodium intake. Perhaps you could use those types of foods less often, or in smaller quantities. Watching your fat and sodium can be a real challenge at certain meals or snacks. See Section 4 for ideas on healthful snacks, desserts, and tips for eating out.

Recipe Work Sheet

Is your favorite recipe high in fat or sodium? Write your recipe below and check pages 40 and 65 of this bulletin for ideas on how you might modify your recipe to reduce fat and sodium.

Ingredients	Amounts	Changes

Preparation	Changes

Try this recipe. It's low in fat and sodium.

Chili Bean Dip

About 1-1/3 cups
Per tablespoon:

Calories	15	Cholesterol	0
Total fat	Trace	Sodium	55 milligrams
Saturated fatty acids.	Trace		

Kidney beans	15-ounce can
Drained bean liquid	3 tablespoons
Vinegar	1 tablespoon
Chili powder	1 teaspoon
Ground cumin	1/8 teaspoon
Onion, grated	2 teaspoons
Parsley, chopped	2 teaspoons

1. Drain kidney beans; save liquid.
2. Place drained beans, bean liquid, vinegar, and seasonings in blender. Blend until smooth.
3. Remove mixture from blender. Stir in onion and parsley.
4. Chill thoroughly.
5. Serve with crisp vegetable sticks.

NOTES:

Food Facts for Older Adults

Special Advice for Older Adults

2

As you age, health conditions may limit what you can eat. This can make eating a balanced diet more difficult. You may need to pay more attention to getting adequate nutrients and fluids and to achieving and maintaining a healthy weight. You may also need to consider possible interactions between foods and medications.

Meeting Your Nutrient Needs

Until recently, research on nutritional requirements has focused on younger people. No one really knows enough about how nutritional needs change as people age. Researchers believe you need the same variety of foods as younger people, but different quantities of some nutrients. Furthermore, individual health and level of activity differ widely among the older population. The best strategy is to figure out a balanced approach to eating that fits your general health and preferences. Use the food guide on the next page to help you make food choices for a healthy diet.

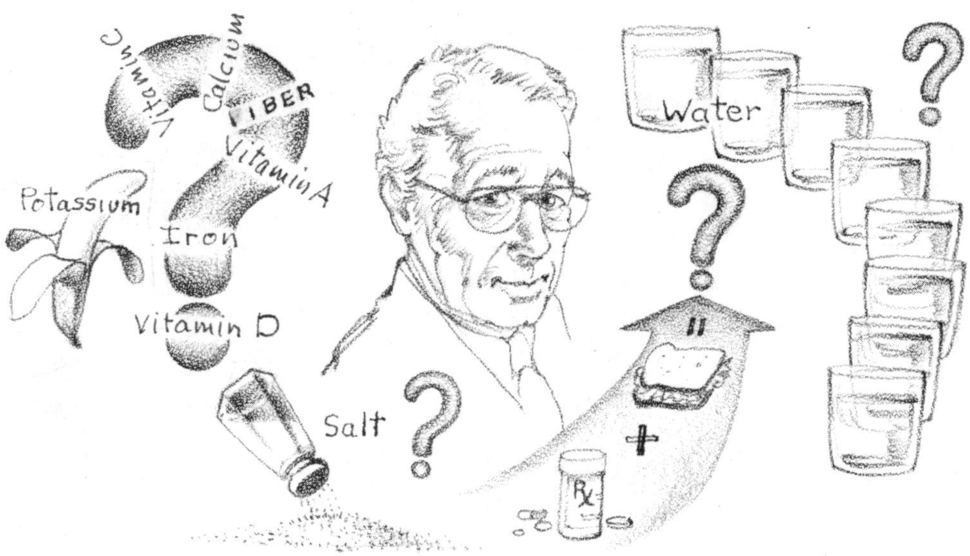

Use the guide below to help you remember what foods and how much to eat each day. Each of the food groups in the three lower levels of the Pyramid supplies specific vitamins and minerals, so it's important to include them all to get the nutrients you need for good health. Try to have at least the lowest number of suggested servings from each of these food groups every day. The lowest number of servings, with modest amounts of fat and sweets, provides about 1,600 calories—right for many older women. Older men need somewhat more (see chart on next page). But remember, individual needs vary, depending on your body size, health, and how active you are. If you need more food, eat more from each of these food groups, and go easy on foods from the fats, oils, and sweets group.

A Guide to Daily Food Choices

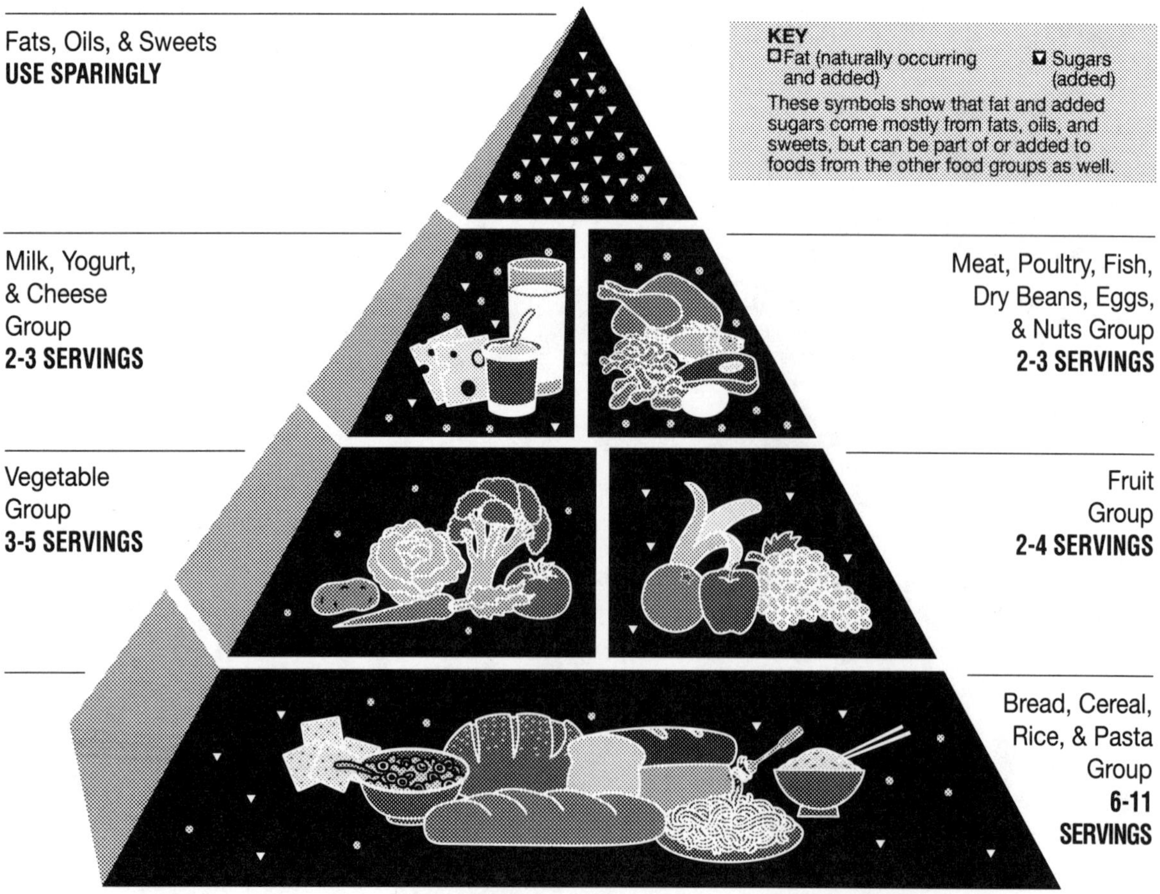

Source: U.S. Department of Agriculture/U.S. Department of Health and Human Services

What counts as 1 serving?

Breads, Cereals, Rice, and Pasta
1 slice of bread
1/2 cup of cooked rice or pasta
1/2 cup of cooked cereal
1 ounce of ready-to-eat cereal

Fruits
1 piece of fruit or melon wedge
3/4 cup of juice
1/2 cup of canned fruit
1/4 cup of dried fruit

Vegetables
1/2 cup of chopped raw or cooked vegetables
1 cup of leafy raw vegetables

Milk, Yogurt, and Cheese
1 cup of milk or yogurt
1-1/2 to 2 ounces of cheese

Meat, Poultry, Fish, Dry Beans, Eggs, and Nuts
2-1/2 to 3 ounces of cooked lean meat, poultry, or fish
Count 1/2 cup of cooked beans or 1 egg or 2 tablespoons of peanut butter as 1 ounce of lean meat (about 1/3 serving)

Fats, Oils, and Sweets
LIMIT CALORIES FROM THESE
especially if you need to lose weight

The amount you eat might be more than one serving. For example, a dinner portion of spaghetti would count as two or three servings of pasta.

Suggested numbers of servings for older adults

Bread group	***6-9**
Vegetable group	***3-4**
Fruit group	***2-3**
Milk group	**2**
Meat group	**2**

*Lower numbers of servings are suggested for older women. The higher numbers are suggested for older men.

A Closer Look at Fat and Added Sugars

The small tip of the Pyramid shows fats, oils, and sweets. These are foods such as salad dressings, cream, butter, margarine, sugars, soft drinks, candies, and sweet desserts. Alcoholic beverages are also part of this group. These foods provide calories but few vitamins and minerals. Most people should go easy on foods from this group.

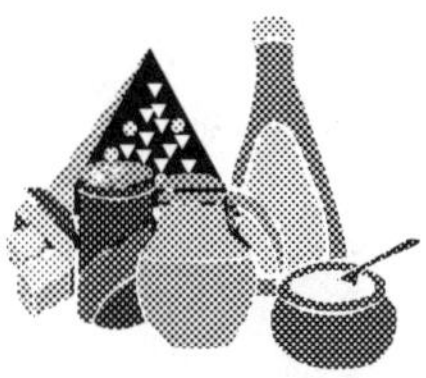

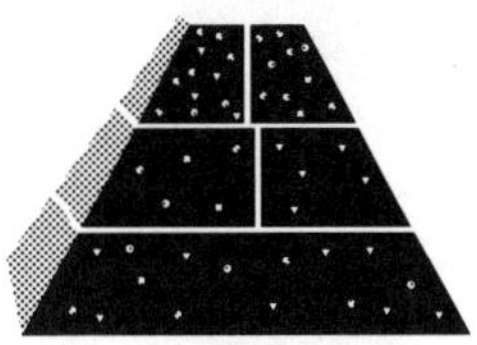

Some fat or sugar symbols are shown in the other food groups. That's to remind you that some foods in these groups can also be high in fat and added sugars, such as cheese or ice cream from the milk group, or french fries from the vegetable group. When choosing foods for a healthful diet, consider the fat and added sugars in your choices from all the food groups, not just fats, oils, and sweets from the Pyramid tip.

DID YOU KNOW???

Learning to estimate serving sizes can be helpful in following the guide to food choices on the previous pages. Here are some typical portion sizes:

- a 1/4-inch-thick slice of cooked lean meat or poultry measuring about 3 x 4 inches weighs about 2 ounces.
- a 3-ounce, cooked, lean hamburger patty starts out as 4 ounces or 1/4 pound of raw meat. The cooked patty will measure about 3 inches across and about 1/2 inch thick, about the size of the palm of a woman's hand, or the size of a large mayonnaise jar lid.
- a 1-inch cube of hard cheese, like Cheddar or swiss, weighs about 1/2 ounce.
- a cooked chicken breast half, without skin, weighs about 3 ounces.

Of Special Interest for Older Adults—Calcium and Vitamin D

All nutrients are important for good health at any age, but some that have been mentioned in the news lately have special importance for older adults. For example, inadequate calcium has been linked to osteoporosis, a condition in which bones become weak and brittle. The exact cause of osteoporosis is not known. Several nutrients in addition to calcium are involved.

However, many scientists believe that women particularly need to get adequate amounts of calcium throughout life. Milk, yogurt, cheese, and other dairy products are the best sources of calcium. Some dark-green leafy vegetables, canned fish eaten with the bones (canned sardines and salmon), and tofu also provide calcium.

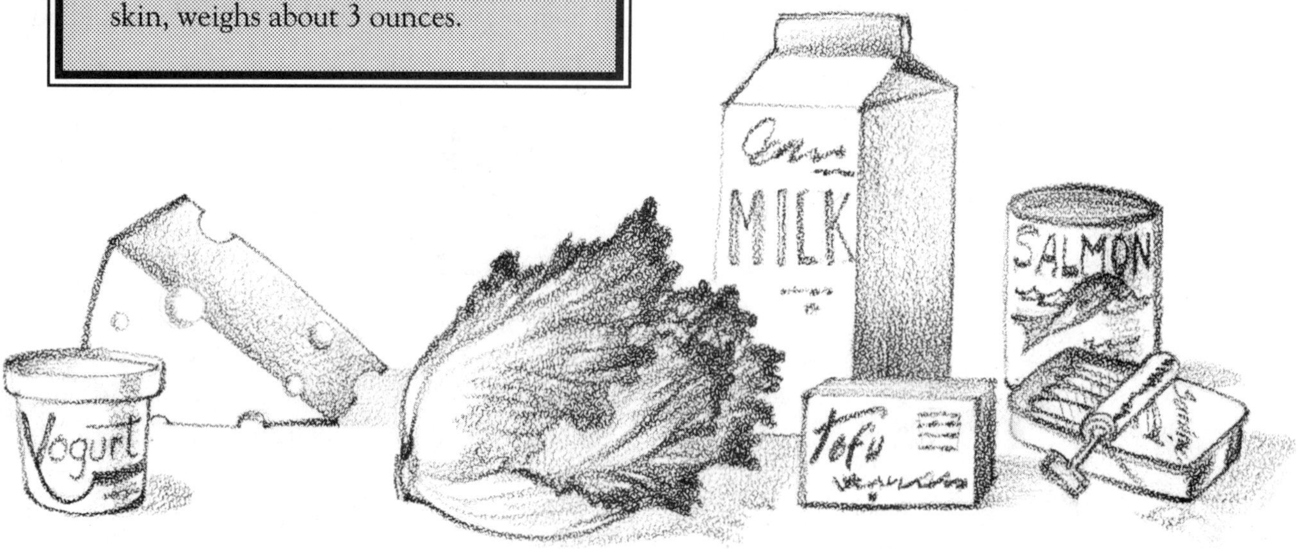

To absorb calcium, your body needs vitamin D. Vitamin D is added to most fluid milk; it can also be made by your skin when exposed to sunlight. Dietary supplements of vitamin D are usually not necessary. Your doctor or dietitian should advise you on your need for additional vitamin D. If they recommend supplements, they should tell you how much you should take. Generally, vitamin D supplements should not exceed the U.S. Recommended Daily Allowance (U.S. RDA) of 400 International Units (IU) per day, because continued use of high doses is harmful. (U.S. RDA's are nutrient standards developed for food product labels by the U.S. Government.)

In addition to getting adequate calcium and vitamin D, it's important to note that moderate exercise that places weight on your bones, such as walking, helps maintain and may even increase bone density and strength in older adults.

Who's at Risk for Osteoporosis?

Anyone can get osteoporosis, but women are at greatest risk, especially white women who are thin, fair-skinned, and small in build. Aging itself, extreme immobility, and genetics, as well as smoking and drinking alcoholic beverages, are believed to contribute to risk for osteoporosis. Loss of calcium from the bones increases in women after menopause, when levels of the hormone estrogen decrease. Estrogen replacement therapy can be prescribed by a doctor to help decrease bone loss after menopause. Because estrogens may have negative side effects in some women, the decision to take estrogen should be made by each woman with the help of her doctor.

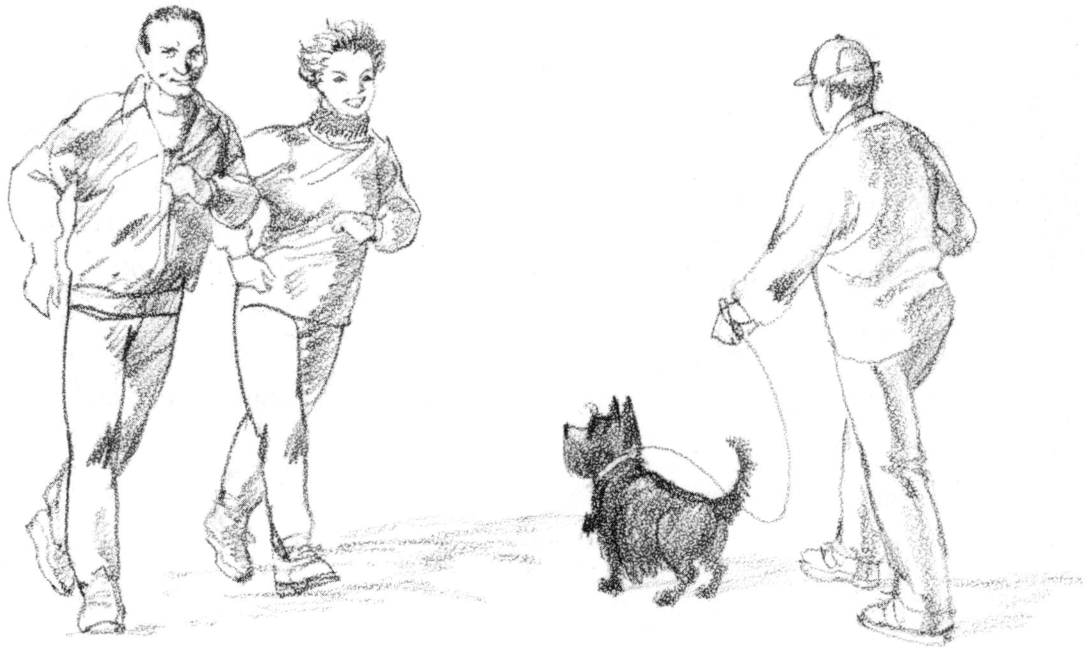

How To Get Enough Calcium If You Don't Drink Milk

Milk is the most obvious and popular source of both calcium and vitamin D, but some people don't drink it and need to consider other ways to get calcium.

Some people have trouble digesting lactose, the sugar occurring naturally in milk. **If you have trouble digesting milk**—

- Drink milk that has had lactase added or add it yourself. Lactase is an enzyme that breaks down milk sugar. It can be purchased at many drug stores.
- Drink only a small amount of milk at a time.
- Eat yogurt or cheese. Lactose has been partially broken down in these foods.
- Try cooked foods made with milk such as soups, puddings, or custards.

If you don't like milk, eat more of other foods with calcium, such as—

- foods made with milk or cheese.
- tofu, a soy product that is sometimes made with calcium sulfate (check the label); 1/2 cup (4 ounces) of tofu made with calcium sulfate has about the same amount of calcium, protein, and fat as 1 cup of whole milk.
- dark-green leafy vegetables, such as kale, collards, and broccoli.
- tortillas made with cornmeal that is fortified with calcium; label may state that the cornmeal is processed with lime, or may list the cornmeal as "masa harina."
- canned or dried fish with edible bones, such as salmon and sardines.

Should You Take a Vitamin Supplement?

Thirty-seven percent of American adults take a daily multivitamin pill. Some even take extra vitamins and minerals as well, especially vitamin C. Yet most of these supplements are unnecessary for people of any age. A well-balanced diet should provide all of your nutritional needs. High doses of some vitamins, such as A and D, can be harmful. Large amounts of some supplements can upset the natural balance of nutrients normally maintained by the body. Large doses, called megavitamins, containing 10 to 100 times the RDA for a vitamin or mineral, can act like drugs, with potentially serious results.

While researchers continue to learn more about how nutrient requirements change during aging, eating a balanced diet containing foods from each food group (listed on the table on page 17 of this section) is the best approach to getting the nutrients you need. Supplements may be beneficial for people who cannot eat a balanced diet or who do not eat enough food, or people who take medicines that interact with nutrients. Before you decide to take a nutritional supplement, discuss it with your doctor or dietitian. If you have specific health problems, or likes and dislikes that greatly limit your food choices, consult a registered dietitian (R.D.) for help in planning the best diet for you.

Drink Enough Fluids

The sense of thirst declines with age, so older people may not drink enough water and other fluids. Sometimes people intentionally drink less to avoid going to the bathroom often. But if you aren't getting enough fluids you can become dehydrated, especially during hot weather.

Drinking plenty of fluids is important to help your body flush out wastes—it's worth a few more trips to the bathroom. Most adults should drink at least eight glasses of water a day. This water can come from any beverage—juice, coffee, tea, milk, or soft drinks—as well as from soup. However, the caffeine in coffee and other drinks may increase your urge to urinate. The sugar in regular soft drinks is an added source of calories you may not need. Plain water, unsweetened fruit juices, and low-fat milk are better choices. Or, for a refreshing carbonated drink, mix fruit juice with club soda or seltzer water. To make plain water more appealing, try it chilled with a twist of lemon or lime.

What About Constipation?

Constipation bothers many older adults. The frequency of bowel movements among healthy people varies from three a day to three a week. Know what is normal for you and avoid relying on laxatives. Drinking enough fluids; eating plenty of fruits, vegetables, and whole-grain products for fiber; and exercising regularly can help with this condition.

Prevention of constipation is the best approach:

- Eat foods with dietary fiber, such as whole-wheat breads and cereals, fruits, and vegetables every day.
- Drink plenty of liquids.
- Exercise regularly.
- Go to the bathroom when you feel the need. Don't delay.

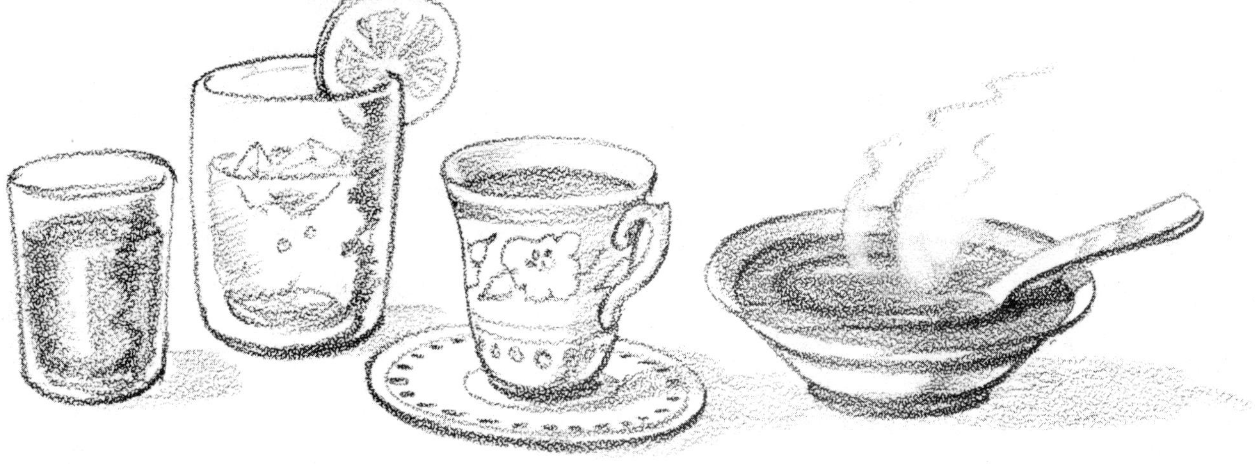

Facts About Fiber

Dietary fiber (sometimes called "roughage") is the part of plant foods that humans can't digest. The fiber passes through the intestines, forming bulk for the stool. There are two major types of fiber—insoluble and soluble. Each has different health benefits, so both are needed in the diet. Insoluble fiber is most often found in whole-grain products, such as whole-wheat bread and cereals, fruits and vegetables with their peels, and dry beans and peas. Insoluble fiber helps prevent constipation. Diets high in insoluble fiber and low in fat may also reduce your risk of colon cancer.

Soluble fiber is found in fruits, vegetables, dry beans and peas, and some cereal products such as oatmeal, oat bran, and rice bran. Some research indicates that diets that are low in fat and saturated fat and rich in soluble fiber may help reduce blood cholesterol levels.

How Much Fiber Should You Eat?

It isn't clear yet exactly how much fiber you should eat each day. Some health experts have suggested that an increase to a range of 20 to 30 grams is a good idea. That's about twice what the average adult eats now. Because plant foods differ in the types and amounts of fiber they contain, it's a good idea to eat different kinds of foods rich in fiber. You can get about 20 grams of fiber if you eat three servings of whole-grain foods, two to three servings of fruit, and three to four servings of vegetables daily. You don't need to take fiber supplements or sprinkle bran on all your foods.

Rx For FIBER [illegible] M.D.

Some choices:

3 servings a day of vegetables	Broccoli spears, corn, potato, and kidney beans
2 servings a day of fruit	Pears, apples, bananas, figs, and oranges
3 servings a day of whole-grain products	Whole-wheat bread, oatmeal, whole-grain cereals

Five Quick Tips To Increase Fiber in Your Diet:

1. Try a whole-grain breakfast cereal, hot or cold. It doesn't have to be 100-percent bran—look for a cereal with at least 2 grams of dietary fiber per serving.
2. Choose baked goods made with whole grains, such as corn muffins; cracked wheat bread; graham crackers; oatmeal bread or muffins; and whole-wheat, pumpernickel or rye breads, rolls, and bagels.
3. Eat fresh fruit or stewed fruit—an orange, half a grapefruit, prunes, or apricots—instead of drinking fruit juice.
4. Eat fruits and vegetables with their peels—apples, pears, peaches, potatoes, or summer squash.
5. Add cooked or canned dry beans, split peas, and lentils to your favorite soups, stews, and salads.

If you're not used to eating foods with fiber, increase fiber gradually to avoid gas or cramping. Be sure to drink enough water or other fluids when you eat more high-fiber foods.

Are You Getting Enough Fiber In Your Diet?

How often do you eat—	Seldom or never	1 to 2 times a week	3 to 5 times a week	Almost daily
1. Three or more servings of breads and cereals made with whole grains?	☐	☐	☐	☐
2. Starchy vegetables such as potatoes, corn, peas, or dishes made with dry beans or peas?	☐	☐	☐	☐
3. Several servings of other vegetables?	☐	☐	☐	☐
4. Whole fruit with skins and/or seeds (berries, apples, pears, etc.)?	☐	☐	☐	☐

The best answer is ALMOST DAILY. Whole-grain products, fruits, and vegetables provide fiber. Eating a variety of these foods daily will provide you with adequate fiber, both soluble and insoluble types.

Avoiding Problems When Medications and Foods Don't Mix

Many older adults take several medications, both prescription and over-the-counter types. It's important to find out from your doctor or pharmacist if these medicines are affected by food or beverages. Some medicines must be taken with meals, while others work better on an empty stomach. Some medicines may have serious or unpleasant side effects or may not work as well if taken in combination with certain foods or alcoholic beverages. Writing out a schedule for your meals and medicines can help you take your medicines properly and get adequate nutrition—both are important to your health.

Ask your doctor or pharmacist if there are special instructions about diet and if there are foods you should avoid when taking your medicine. You may need special advice about diet and—

- diuretics and other high blood pressure medicines,
- some antibiotics,
- some pain relievers,
- some antidepressants,
- anticoagulants (drugs for blood thinning),
- antacids.

Do You Take Medicines Properly?

When you get a new prescription medicine, be sure you understand **when** to take it, **how much** to take, **how long** to take it, and what **to do** if you miss a dose.

Tell your doctor about any other medicines you may be taking, including those prescribed by other doctors, over-the-counter medicines, and any vitamins or other supplements.

Ask whether there are foods or over-the-counter medicines you should **not** take with your new prescription.

Contact your doctor or pharmacist right away if you experience any side effects. If you are taking several medicines for long periods, ask your doctor every once in a while if you should still be taking all of them. Don't stop taking any prescribed medicines without consulting your doctor.

Make sure you understand the name of the drug and directions printed on the container. Ask your pharmacist to use large type if necessary. If child-proof containers are hard to handle, ask for easy-to-open containers.

Discard old prescription medicines and expired over-the-counter drugs. Never take drugs that were prescribed for a friend or relative, even though your symptoms may be the same.

Planning a Menu Using the Food Guide

The sample menu on the next page shows how you might use the Food Guide Pyramid on page 16 of this section.

The 1,600-calorie menu includes the lower numbers of servings from the food groups, and the 2,400-calorie menu includes the higher numbers of servings shown in the table on page 17. Jelly, margarine, sherbet, and lemonade are extras, from the Fats, Oils, and Sweets group. Listed below are nutrient values for the two menus:

	1,600 Calorie Menu	2,400 Calorie Menu
Total fat, grams	46	75
% of calories	26	28
Saturated fat, grams	18	24
% of calories	10	9
Cholesterol, mg	185	235
Sodium, mg	2,190	3,010
Dietary fiber, grams	18	30

ASK YOURSELF...

- Do I eat foods from all the food groups each day?
- Am I getting enough calcium-rich foods?
- Do I need to take a vitamin supplement, or can I add foods to my diet that will provide me with the nutrients I need?
- Have I discussed the vitamins I take with my doctor or a dietitian?
- How much fluid do I drink each day?
- Are these fluids high in calories?
- Do I know how all of the medications I am taking interact with foods or drinks?

Menu

1,600 calories		2,400 calories
BREAKFAST		
1/2 medium	Grapefruit	1/2 medium
2 slices	Whole-wheat toast	2 slices
1 tsp.	Margarine, soft	2 tsp.
None	Jelly	1 tbsp.
1 cup	Milk, skim	1 cup
LUNCH		
6 fl. oz.	Vegetable juice, no salt added	6 fl. oz.
	Luncheon salad:	
1 oz.	Turkey	2 oz.
1 oz.	Ham	1 oz.
1-1/2 oz.	Swiss cheese	1-1/2 oz.
1-1/2 cups	Mixed greens	1-1/2 cups
1 tbsp.	French dressing, low calorie	1-1/2 tbsp.
2 small	Corn muffins	3 small
1 medium	Peach, fresh	2 medium
DINNER		
3 oz.	Sirloin steak, broiled (lean only)	3 oz.
1/2 cup	Yellow corn, fresh or frozen	1 cup
1/2 cup	Stewed tomatoes, no salt added	1/2 cup
1 small	Whole-grain roll	2 small
1 tsp.	Margarine, soft	1 tsp.
1/2 cup	Lime sherbet	1/2 cup
As desired	Coffee, tea, or water	As desired
SNACKS		
None	Peanut butter sandwich	1 sandwich
	2 slices of whole-wheat bread	
	2 tbsp. of peanut butter	
	2 tsp. of jelly	
3 squares	Graham crackers	None
8 fl. oz.	Lemonade	8 fl. oz.

Food Facts for Older Adults

Making Healthy Food Choices When You Shop and Cook

3

Many older adults who once cooked and shopped for families now find they must adjust their shopping and preparation to fit the appetite of one or two people. Others find themselves on their own in the kitchen or supermarket for the first time. Most are becoming more concerned about calories, fat, and sodium in their diets. Here are some tips on how to manage in an increasingly complex marketplace.

Use Food Labels

Food labels are the best source of specific information about the foods you buy and eat. They can help you choose between similar products. Here is what you need to know:

Ingredients are listed in order by weight, from the largest amount to the least amount.

Check the ingredient list for ingredients you may want to limit, such as salt, saturated fats, or sugars, or those you want to increase, such as whole grains in baked products.

Nutrition information lists calories, protein, carbohydrates, fat, sodium, and various vitamins and minerals contained in a serving of the food. Saturated fat, cholesterol, and dietary fiber may also be listed. Amounts of vitamins and minerals are listed as percentages of the U.S. Recommended Daily Allowances (U.S. RDA's), nutrient standards developed for food product labels by the U.S. Government.

DID YOU KNOW???

Food ingredient statements on labels may list different forms of the same ingredient separately. For example, a product may list several forms of sugar, such as sugar, corn syrup, honey, or molasses. If several forms are listed, the product probably is high in sugar.

Some Hints on Using the Nutrition Label:

Check the nutrition information for:

- **Serving size** - Is it the amount you usually eat?

- **Amounts of fat and sodium per serving—** Is the fat or sodium high? For a point of reference, compare the amount per serving of the product to the total amounts suggested per day:

  Fat: Suggested amount is 30 percent of daily calories--
  53 grams per day for 1,600-calorie diets
  80 grams per day for 2,400-calorie diets
  For example, a food that provides 20 grams of fat would provide over one-third of the day's fat in a 1,600-calorie diet.

  Sodium: 2,400 mg or less per day is suggested by some health authorities.

- **Amounts of vitamins or minerals** of special interest to you, such as calcium. Look for foods that have a significant amount of the vitamin or mineral (10 percent or more of the U.S. RDA), but not too many calories.

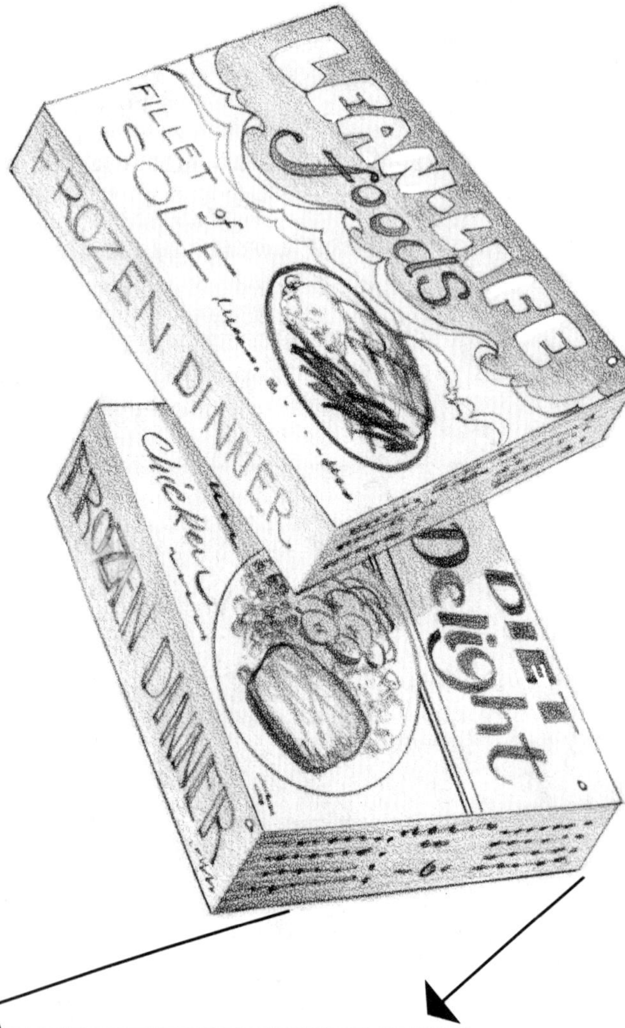

Nutrition Information Per Serving
Serving size: 11.25 oz.
Servings per container: 1

Calories	240	Polyunsaturated Fat	LESS THAN 1g
Protein	20g	Saturated Fat	1g
Carbohydrate	36g	Cholesterol	45mg
Fat	2g	Sodium	400mg

Is It Fresh?

Many products now have **open dating,** which provides information on freshness in several ways:

- the **pull-by** or **sell-by** date tells you when the product should be sold or taken off the shelves by the grocery store.

- **best used by** date is typically found on bakery goods and packaged cereals—it's the last day the product can be expected to be at its peak quality.

- **expiration** or **use by** date, usually on refrigerated products, is the last date the food should be used.

- **pack date** is the date the food was processed or packaged and is usually found on foods like canned goods that have a long shelf life. Be sure not to buy any bulging or leaking cans. The food is unsafe.

These dates tell you how long you can store and use the product. This will be helpful if you can't shop often.

Food Shopping, Dietary Guidelines Style

Whether you are age 7 or 70, you need a variety of foods from each of the food groups. There are many choices available in today's typical supermarket. Here are some food choices that will help you get the variety you need while watching your fat, cholesterol, and sodium intake. Try a few the next time you shop.

Breads, cereals, rice, and pasta:

- whole-wheat, rye, pumpernickel, mixed grain, and enriched breads and rolls, bagels, and english muffins
- whole-grain crackers, such as graham crackers, wheat crackers, and rice cakes
- whole-grain breakfast cereals
- plain rice, pasta (cook with less salt)

Fruits:

- fresh fruit
- canned fruit, in juice rather than heavy syrup
- canned or frozen fruit juice, unsweetened

> ***DID YOU KNOW???***
>
> You can ask the grocer to divide packages of fresh vegetables or eggs and cut smaller portions of meat for you. You don't have to buy more than you can use.

More shopping ideas . . .

Vegetables:

- fresh leafy vegetables and other vegetables (use within a few days)
- carrots, potatoes, onions (will keep longer)
- frozen vegetables without sauce
- canned vegetables, tomato sauces, and soups; try those with reduced sodium, or no salt added, if available
- dry beans or split peas; canned beans; bean and pea soups.

Meat, poultry, fish:

- fresh, well-trimmed, lean meats—beef round, loin, sirloin, chuck arm; pork loin, roasts, and chops; leg of lamb—(1/2 pound trimmed boneless raw meat will make about two 3-ounce cooked servings)
- for leaner ground beef, ask the butcher to trim fat off and grind a piece of beef round steak
- fresh chicken, turkey parts; boneless, skinless breasts or thighs
- fresh or plain frozen fish; tuna fish canned in water
- eggs (you may want to buy only a half-dozen)
- peanut butter

Milk, yogurt, cheese:

- lowfat (2 percent or 1 percent) or skim milk
- lowfat or nonfat yogurt, plain or flavored
- part-skim and lowfat cheeses such as mozzarella, ricotta, cottage cheese
- frozen yogurt or ice milk

Spreads and seasonings:

- margarine, with liquid vegetable oil listed as the first ingredient
- vegetable oils, such as canola, olive, corn, and soybean oils, for cooking and salad dressings
- low-calorie mayonnaise and salad dressings
- salt-free herb blends for seasoning

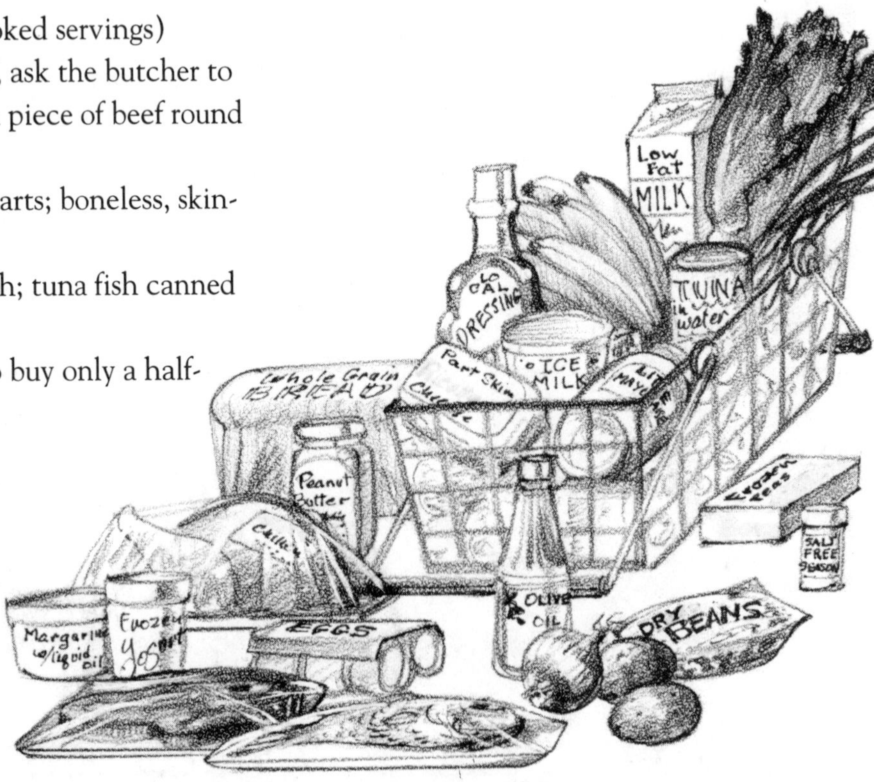

New on the Market — Lower Fat, Lower Sodium, Lower Sugar Products

Many new foods are available to help you choose a diet that is low in fat, sugars, and sodium. One no longer has to go to the dietetic section of the supermarket to find fruits canned in juice instead of heavy syrup, canned vegetables with no salt added, and soups with reduced sodium content. Even frozen dinners come in varieties that are low in fat and sodium. Some manufacturers also have reformulated their baked products and frozen dairy desserts to produce "ice creams", cookies, cakes, and pastries that are nearly fat and cholesterol free.

Low-calorie sweeteners are widely used to sweeten soft drinks, fruit punches, puddings, gelatin desserts, yogurts, frozen dairy desserts, and many other foods. Low-calorie, low-cholesterol fat substitutes processed from egg white and skim milk proteins are used in gourmet-style frozen dairy desserts and may be used in other cold products, such as salad dressings, sour cream, and cheese spreads. Food scientists are developing other heat-stable substances that may partially substitute for fat in frying.

Are fat and sugar substitutes safe? The Food and Drug Administration (FDA) must approve food additives and novel ingredients such as fat and sugar substitutes before they can be used in foods. If you have questions about the safety of a food additive or ingredient, contact the FDA Consumer Affairs Office on the resource list included in this bulletin. As always, moderation in use of these products is the best advice. It is not necessary to use products containing fat or sugar substitutes to have a healthy diet.

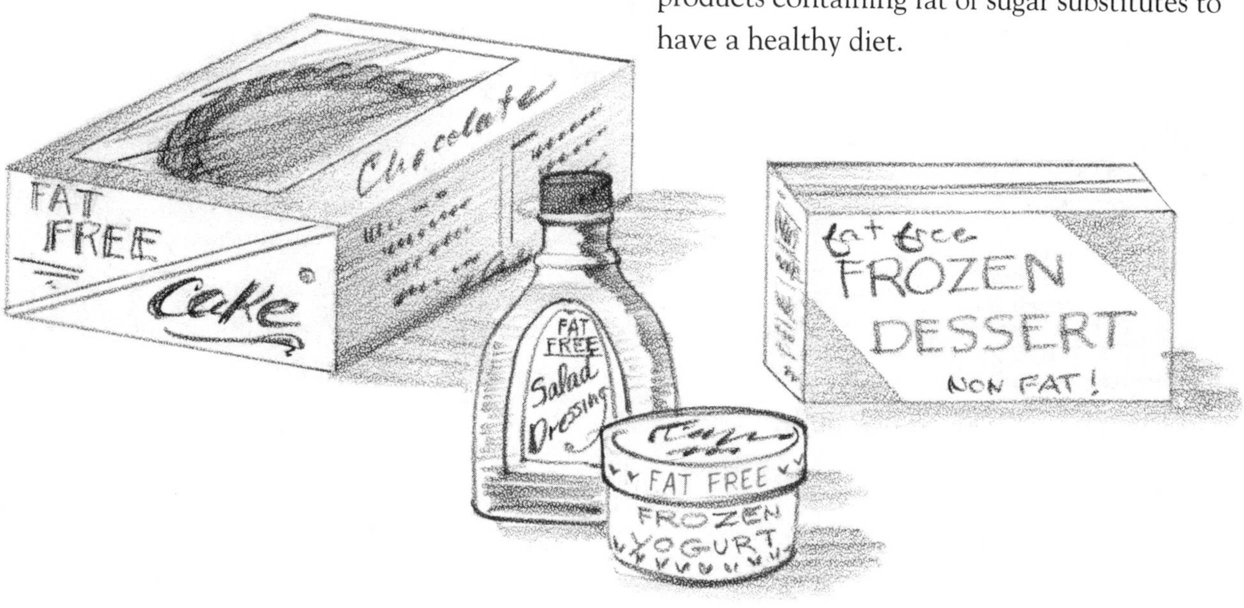

What's To Eat?—Quick and Easy Meals for One or Two People

Here are some ideas to get you started on making easy and nutritious meals for one or two people:

- Cook once and eat twice, or even three times. Cook a small roast; eat one portion now and freeze additional portions to mix with vegetables for quick soups, stews, or chili.

- Buy frozen vegetables in 1-pound bags. Cook what you need for single or double servings or mix several kinds for an interesting vegetable medley.

- Keep several kinds of pasta on hand. Many cook quickly. Pasta makes an attractive side dish, or it can be used as a base for stews or topped with a lowfat sauce. Make single servings or cook extra to add to soups or casseroles. Mix with vegetables and a lowfat dressing for pasta salad.

- Try a baked fruit for dessert—one or two servings cook quickly in a microwave oven, or bake the fruit along with another food prepared in the oven. Serve warm, with a dash of cinnamon or nutmeg.

Dinner's in the Freezer!

Frozen dinners and entrees are becoming staples in many one- and two-person households. They offer convenient, quick-cooking, tasty meals with little waste and clean-up. Even if you don't use them regularly, it's nice to have one or two on hand for those times when you just don't feel like cooking. Here are some hints for choosing frozen dinners and entrees and using these foods as part of a healthy diet:

❶ **Read the label.** Use the nutrition label, the ingredient label, and even the name and the picture of the product to see what you are getting.

- Read the ingredient label to see what ingredients are present and in what amounts. Products containing cream sauces, cheese, and ground meat are likely to be higher in fat than products made with lean cuts of meat, vegetables, and broth. Oriental-style products containing soy sauce or teriyaki sauce are likely to be higher in sodium.

- Read the nutrition label for the calories, fat, sodium, and other nutrients per serving of the product. Many frozen dinners and entrees are relatively high in sodium or fat, even the low- calorie types.

- When you look at the nutrition label, think how the amount of fat or sodium compares to the amounts that are right for you for the whole day. Also think about what else you will be eating at that meal or that day that can help you moderate your total fat and sodium intake. If you choose a high- fat or high-sodium entree for one meal, make an effort to choose foods low in fat or sodium for the next meal.

- The name and the picture can also provide clues to product composition. For example, "beef dinner" will generally have more beef than "beef with vegetables in sauce." The picture on the package should show the contents of the product too.

❷ **Decide what else to eat with the frozen dinner or entree.** Most frozen dinners or entrees provide only 300 to 500 calories. They usually include about 2 to 2-1/2 ounces of meat, 1 to 1-1/2 servings of vegetables, and less than 1 serving of grain products such as rice or noodles. Large serving types—"for big appetites"—provide somewhat more. If the product is your main meal of the day, you'll probably want to eat something else with it.

Try these easy, healthy additions:

- a large whole-grain roll
- a small salad or 1/2 cup of frozen vegetables (microwave it along with your dinner in a covered container with 2 teaspoons of water)
- milk as your beverage, or yogurt or milk pudding for dessert
- fresh or canned sliced fruit—which can top the yogurt or pudding

If your frozen dinner or entree is high in fat or sodium, choose lower fat or sodium foods to go with it. Go easy on fatty spreads and dressing, and don't add salt at the table.

❸ **Make your own frozen meals**—it's a great way to use leftovers and save money as well as time. Cook extra when you have time, and divide cooked meat or other main dishes into single portions on a microwave or oven-safe plate. (Plain sliced meat should have a lowfat gravy or other liquid to moisten it.) Add a serving or two of frozen vegetables with 2 teaspoons of water. Cover tightly and freeze promptly. For best quality, use your home-prepared dinners within 2 months.

Focus on Food Safety

Older people are more vulnerable to foodborne illness, so it's important to handle foods safely:

✔Check your food safety practices.

Do you–

- ☐ Always wash hands with warm soapy water before handling food?
- ☐ Thaw frozen foods in the refrigerator, not on the kitchen counter? Or thaw them in the microwave, following the oven manufacturer's directions?
- ☐ Cook raw meats, poultry, fish, and eggs thoroughly?
- ☐ Keep hot foods hot and cold foods cold until serving time?
- ☐ Refrigerate or freeze leftover foods promptly? Don't let perishable foods sit out at room temperature for more than 2 hours.

For answers to your food safety questions, contact:

- a County Extension Home Economist (look in your phone book under county government, Cooperative Extension Service, or your State university)
- USDA's Meat and Poultry Hotline (1-800-535-4555), weekdays, 10-4 Eastern time (in Washington, DC, area, call 202-720-3333)

Food Facts for Older Adults

Maintaining a Healthy Weight

4

Many Americans are overweight. Being overweight can increase your risk for high blood pressure, diabetes, heart disease, and certain cancers. Recent research suggests that people can be a little heavier as they grow older without added risk to health, although just how much heavier is not yet clear. Talk with your doctor to determine if your weight is right for you.

As people age, they usually need fewer calories to maintain a healthy weight. Older people may become less active too. Achieving and maintaining a healthy weight should be an ongoing part of caring for your health. If you need to lose some weight, don't try to lose weight too fast and avoid extreme approaches. Remember, quick weight loss plans often deprive the body of important nutrients and usually don't keep weight off.

Be Physically Active

Physical activity can help reduce and control weight by burning up calories and should be part of a healthy lifestyle at any age. Moderate exercise that places weight on your bones, such as walking, helps maintain and possibly even increases bone strength in older adults—another good reason to exercise. Scientists looking into the benefits of exercise for older adults agree that appropriate exercise improves overall health at any age. Regular exercise can improve the functioning of the heart and lungs, increase strength and flexibility, and contribute to a feeling of well-being.

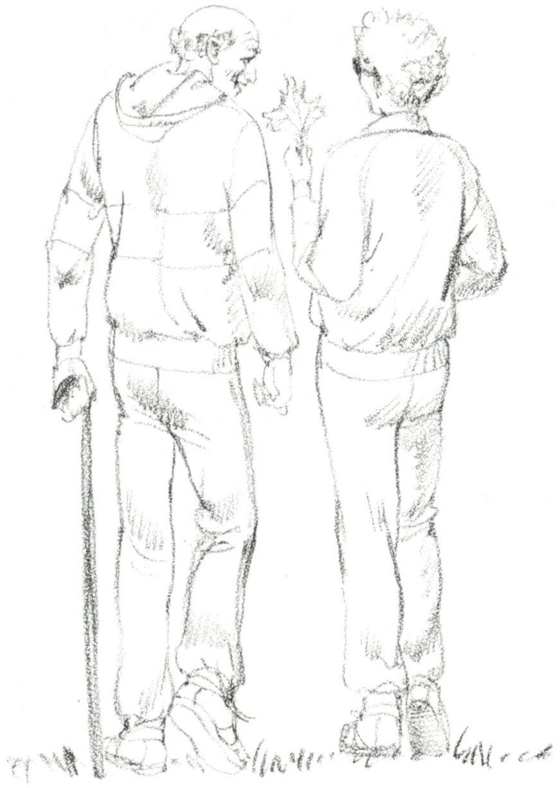

You don't have to jog or do aerobics to benefit from exercise. Any regular physical activity is good. Regular brisk walking is an easy and enjoyable form of exercise that helps control weight, but you will benefit from any form of gentle exercise, even light gardening. Use your common sense to prevent injury when you exercise, and check with your doctor before beginning a vigorous exercise program or if you haven't exercised in a while.

> ***DID YOU KNOW???***
>
> Starchy foods such as breads, cereals, rice, pasta, corn, and potatoes are usually low in fat and provide fiber, as well as vitamins and minerals. Yet many people don't want to eat more breads and potatoes, because they think these foods are fattening. Actually, more calories are likely to come from the fat you put on these foods—butter, sour cream, or gravy—than from the "starch" itself. Eating more starchy foods is a good way to satisfy your appetite while watching your weight. Just go easy on the toppings!

Reduce Calories, Not Vitamins and Minerals

To lose weight you need to reduce the amount of calories you eat. But, you need to do this without giving up important nutrients. A weight-reduction diet will be difficult to follow if you always feel hungry. Choosing lowfat foods allows you to cut calories without sacrificing important vitamins and minerals. For example, 1 cup of skim milk has about the same amount of calcium as 1 cup of whole milk, but only traces of fat and half the number of calories. On the other hand, fatty spreads and dressings, sugary foods such as candy or soft drinks, and alcoholic beverages such as beer, wine, and liquors add calories to your diet but little or no nutrients. Limiting your intake of fats, sweets, and alcoholic beverages will help keep the calories in your diet down, without sacrificing nutrients.

Some Advice About Diet Claims and Dieting

Our society's preoccupation with weight loss has created a multimillion-dollar industry that abounds with diet plans and claims. Some diet plans simply don't work at all, and others are harmful. Always seek the advice of your doctor or dietitian before you begin any special diet.

Beware of diets that—

- make unrealistic promises—for example, dramatic weight loss in a short period of time.
- include fasting.
- eliminate one food group completely or include only one or two food groups.
- have a daily caloric intake that **exceeds** your usual caloric intake.
- do not allow you to have a favorite food on occasion.
- include foods that are expensive or difficult to find.
- require costly fees.
- do not address changing your eating habits.

The **best advice** for weight loss is not contained in any one diet, but simply follows some common sense ideas:

- Consult your doctor.
- Eat a well-balanced diet with a variety of foods from each food group.
- Make a long-term commitment to healthy eating habits.
- Include regular exercise.
- Create or choose a plan that fits your food preferences.
- Remember that radical changes are hard to make. Instead, begin to modify your intake by eating smaller portions and reducing fat, sugar, and, if you drink, alcoholic beverages.

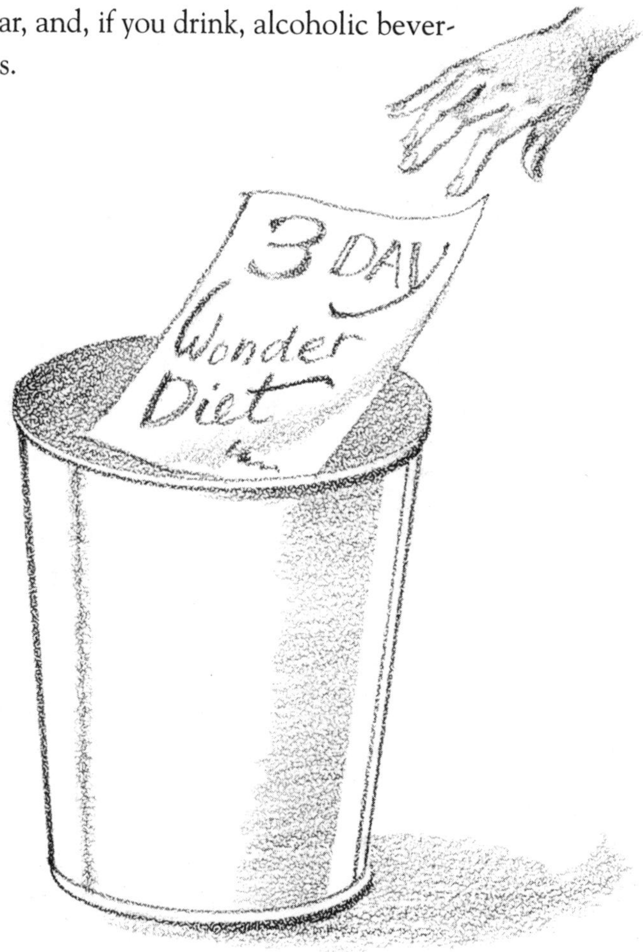

What If I'm Underweight?

Though discussions of diet usually focus on losing weight, some people have trouble maintaining enough weight. This sometimes happens to older people when they find themselves living alone. People who are underweight are often more susceptible to illnesses and don't recover from them as well as others. If you are concerned about weighing too little, try to—

- eat three balanced meals every day, with foods from each food group.
- increase portion sizes of the foods you eat at each meal.
- try new foods and ingredients to perk up your appetite.
- eat when you feel hungry. Keep healthy snacks handy for munching and don't skip meals.
- try milk, cocoa, or soup instead of coffee and tea, which have few calories.
- add milk, cheeses, and crumb toppings to casseroles, soups, stews, or side dishes.

Food Choice Challenges

Some situations pose special challenges for making healthy food choices, especially snacktime, dessert time, and eating out.

Snacking

Americans, in general, are snackers and often substitute snacks for meals because they are quick and easy. Eating too many snacks that are high in sugar, fat, and salt can add calories without giving you important nutrients you need. On the other hand, nutritious snacks can help you get needed nutrients, especially if you find it easier to eat only small amounts of food at meals.

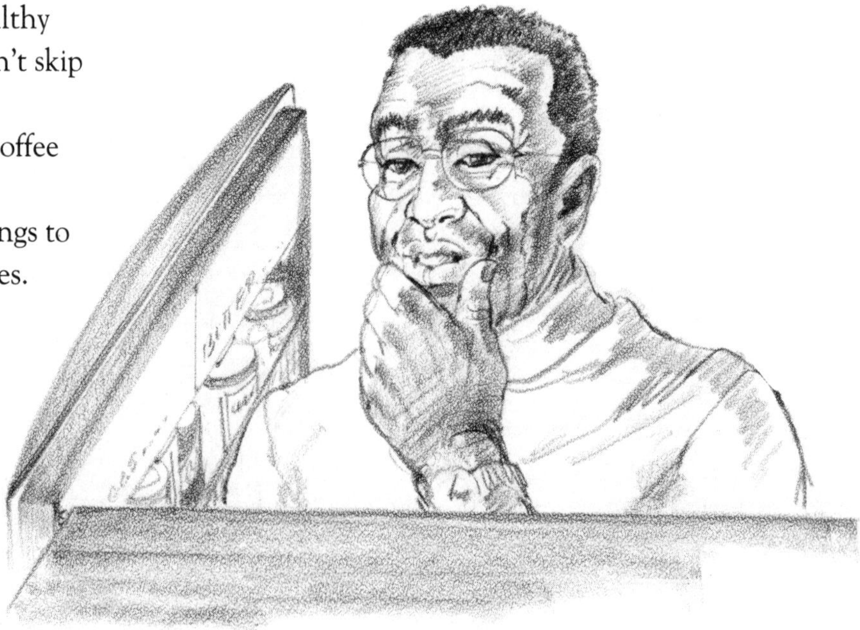

Ten Ideas for Healthy Snacking

1. plain popcorn, without added butter or oil
2. whole-grain crackers
3. unsalted pretzels
4. lowfat yogurt
5. lowfat cheeses and spreads
6. unsweetened fruit juices
7. tomato juice
8. fruit slices with peels (for more fiber)
9. raw vegetable strips and pieces
10. sparkling water flavored with a slice of lemon or lime

Limit the amount of food you eat at snack-time, so you won't be tempted to skip meals. For instance, take several crackers and eat them slowly—don't take a whole box of crackers to munch on. If you need to make your snack a mini-meal, try eating "meal foods"—half a sandwich and a glass of milk or a cup of soup. If you're limiting calories, choose lowfat dairy products and clear soups.

Desserts Can Be Nutritious Too

For many people, desserts are another source of "empty calories"—foods that add a lot of calories without many nutrients. You don't have to cut out desserts; many recipes for baked desserts can be modified to be lower in salt, fat, cholesterol, and sugar. Ingredients with dietary fiber, such as whole grains and dried fruits, can be added too. There are also low-calorie or lower fat substitutes available for ice cream, sour cream, and whipped cream.

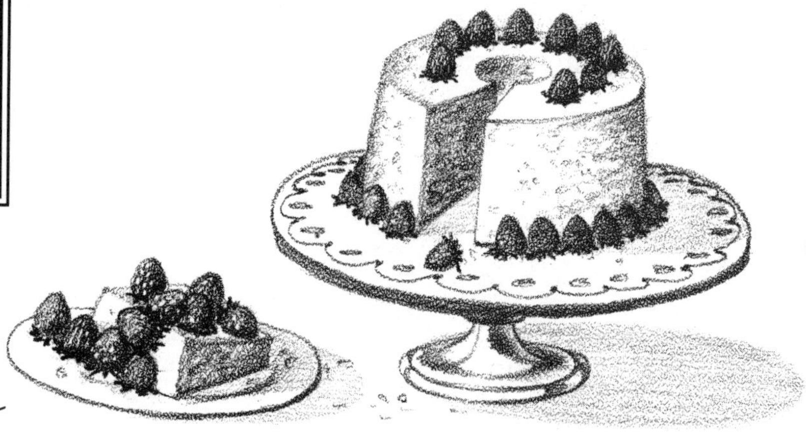

Hints for Reducing Fat, Saturated Fat, Cholesterol, Sugar, and Sodium in Your Baking

FOR...	USE...
whole egg	2 egg whites
whole milk	skim or lowfat milk
sugar	1/2 cup of sugar per cup of flour in cakes 1 tablespoon of sugar per cup of flour in yeast breads Hint: when reducing sugar, add more flavoring, such as vanilla
baking chocolate, 1 oz.	3 tablespoons of cocoa (if fat is needed, use 1 tablespoon or less of oil)
fat	minimum for muffins and quick breads is 1 to 2 tablespoons of fat per cup of flour minimum for cakes is 2 tablespoons of fat per cup of flour Hint: soft drop cookies generally contain less fat than rolled cookies
sodium	1/4 teaspoon of salt per cup of flour in yeast breads; half the amount of salt called for in other baked products 1-1/4 teaspoons of baking powder per cup of flour in muffins, biscuits, waffles 1 teaspoon of baking powder per cup of flour in cakes
sour cream	lowfat sour cream or yogurt
butter	margarine or vegetable oil (total fat will be the same, but saturated fat and cholesterol will be reduced)

Some Tips for Making Desserts More Nutritious:

TRY—

- fruit breads made with whole-wheat flour.
- fresh fruit, baked or broiled, spiced with cinnamon, nutmeg, or mint.
- pudding made with lowfat milk and less sugar.
- unsweetened fresh fruit topped with lowfat yogurt.
- rolled oat toppings for fruit crisps, instead of flour/sugar/butter crumb toppings.
- cookie recipes with less sugar and fat.
- single-crust pies—try a crust made with 1 cup of graham cracker crumbs and 3 tablespoons of soft margarine.
- ice milk, frozen yogurt, sherbets, sorbet, or flavored ices. When you do eat ice cream, try regular varieties rather than the rich super premium types, which are much higher in fat.

DID YOU KNOW???

Sugar means more than just white table sugar. It means all forms of caloric sweeteners, including brown sugar, raw sugar, corn syrup, honey, and molasses. All contain calories but relatively few nutrients. It's okay to enjoy a sweet now and then — but if you're trying to cut calories, go easy.

Eating Better When Eating Out

More and more Americans are eating out, and older Americans are no exception. While you can't control the ingredients in the foods you eat in restaurants, you can choose wisely and eat moderate amounts.

The type of restaurant you eat in will determine what choices you can make. For example, cafeterias and buffets offer a variety of foods but no options for ordering foods prepared as you like. And restaurants offering "all-you-can-eat" tempt you to eat too much! Fast-food restaurants also limit your choices because many items are deep-fat fried or contain a lot of sodium. However, many chains now have salad bars, offering a healthful alternative.

The key strategies to eating healthy in a restaurant are watching serving sizes so you don't overeat, choosing items that are low in fat, and asking for alternatives like lowfat milk and margarine when possible.

Some Tips for Eating Healthy at Restaurants:

- Choose steamed, grilled, stirfried, or baked meats and vegetables.
- Limit the amount of fried foods, heavy sauces, and gravies you eat. Choose tomato-based sauces and soups instead of creamed ones.
- Eat bread and potatoes with only small amounts of butter or margarine.
- Order sauces and salad dressings on the side, when possible, and then add them sparingly.
- When portion choices are available, order small or half portions; if they're not available, eat half and take the rest home.
- Choose vegetable toppings for pizza instead of sausage or extra cheese.
- At the salad bar, limit heavy dressings; go easy on toppings like croutons and cheese and items made with mayonnaise, such as macaroni salad.
- Ask questions about what the menu terms mean if you don't understand them. Some terms can be misleading. If you're unsure, ask how the food is prepared or what the ingredients are.
- Don't be afraid to send something back to the kitchen if it tastes too fatty or salty. After all, you haven't paid for it yet!
- You don't have to skip dessert; split one and you give away half the calories too!

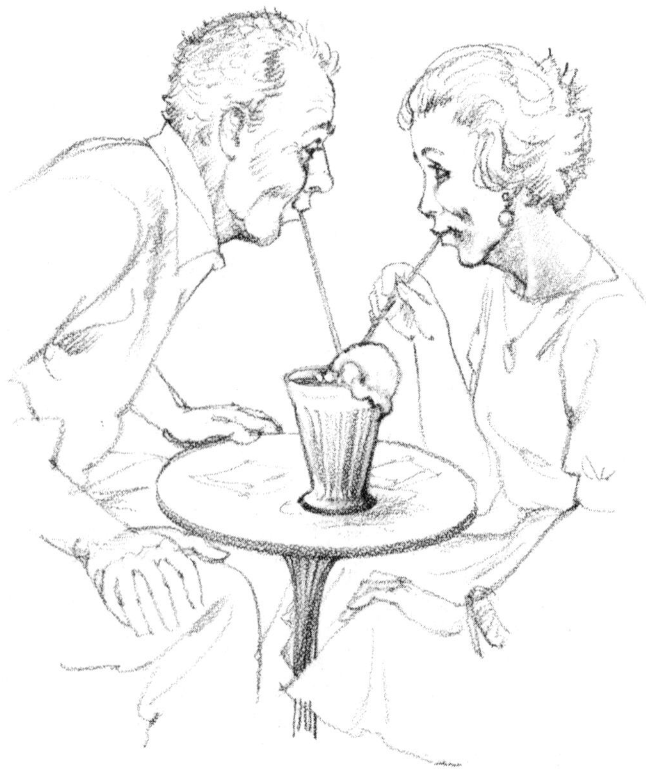

Catching on to Menu Clues

Some terms commonly used in menus can provide clues to higher fat or sodium content.

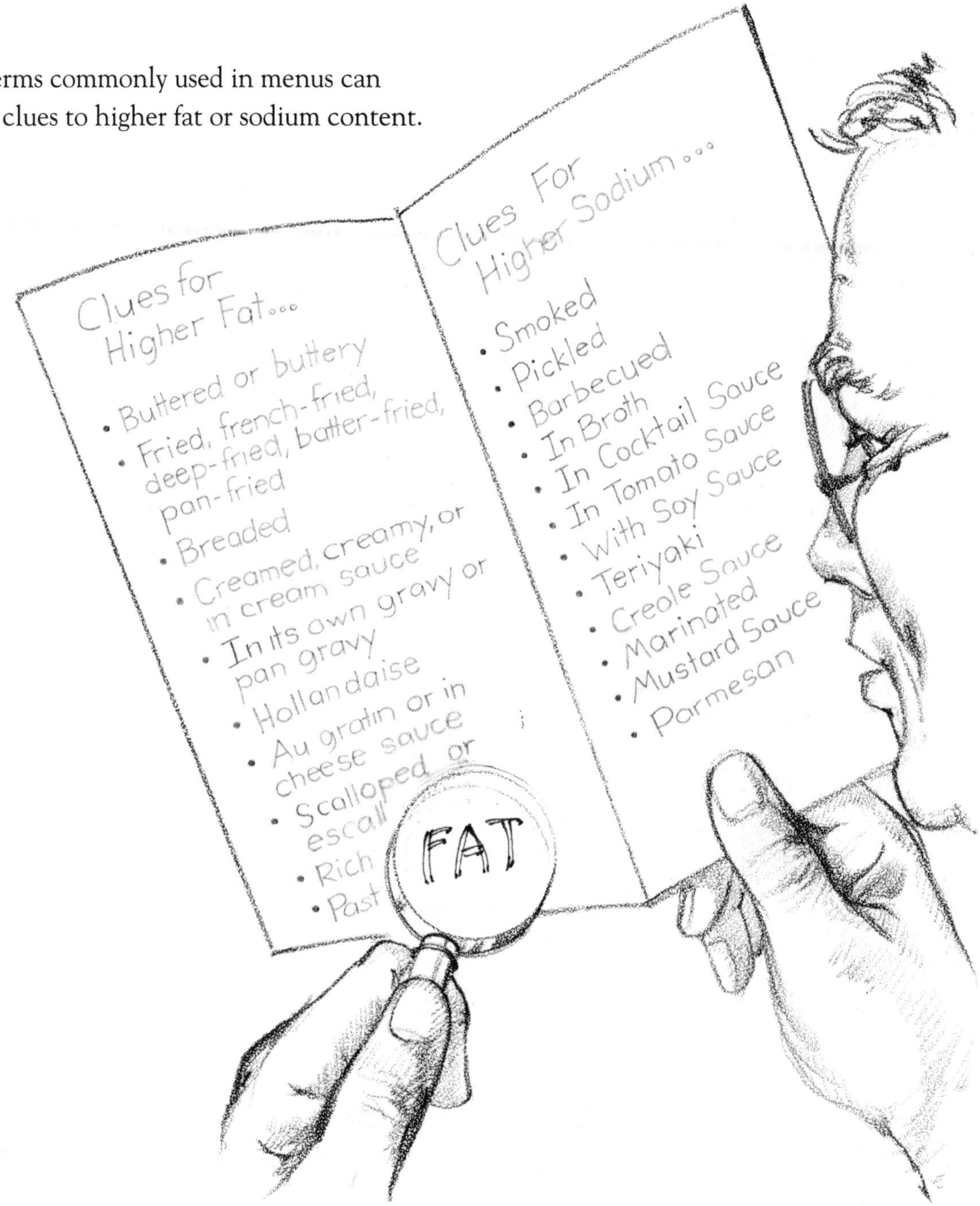

Clues for Higher Fat...
• Buttered or buttery
• Fried, french-fried, deep-fried, batter-fried, pan-fried
• Breaded
• Creamed, creamy, or in cream sauce
• In its own gravy or pan gravy
• Hollandaise
• Au gratin or in cheese sauce
• Scalloped or escall
• Rich
• Past
FAT
Clues For Higher Sodium...
• Smoked
• Pickled
• Barbecued
• In Broth
• In Cocktail Sauce
• In Tomato Sauce
• With Soy Sauce
• Teriyaki
• Creole Sauce
• Marinated
• Mustard Sauce
• Parmesan

Some terms can signal lower fat. Foods that are grilled or broiled, stirfried, roasted, poached, or steamed need less fat in preparation than frying. Few terms guarantee low sodium. Even "fresh" or "homemade" foods can be high in sodium depending on their ingredients and the amounts used.

Fast Food on a Lowfat Budget

You can enjoy fast food without eating too many calories, or too much fat or sodium. Just follow these pointers:

The Main Dish:

- Try hamburgers with one regular patty rather than those with two patties, and plain types rather than those with lots of extras like cheese, bacon, or "special" sauces.
- Order roast beef or grilled chicken for a leaner alternative to most burgers or fried chicken.
- Breaded, deep-fat fried fish and chicken sandwiches (especially those with cheese, tartar sauce, or mayonnaise) have more fat and calories than a plain burger.
- When fixing your sandwich, load up on lettuce, tomato, and onion, **but** limit pickles, mustard, catsup, and other sauces. If you're having fried chicken, remove the skin and some of the breading before you eat. Try broiled chicken as an alternative.

On the Side:

- Skip the fries if you're also ordering a main dish that is deep-fried or made with a sauce or cheese.
- Order a small portion of fries rather than a large one.
- Specify no salt when possible and add a small amount yourself.
- Choose a plain baked potato or mashed potatoes instead of fries, and add butter or margarine and salt sparingly.
- Have a tossed salad instead of fries.
- Ask for a dinner roll instead of a biscuit to limit calories and fat.

Salads:

- Load up on fresh greens, fruits, and vegetables.
- Go easy on the dressings and creamy salads such as potato salad, coleslaw, and macaroni or pasta salads.

Beverages:

- Choose milk, preferably skim or lowfat, instead of a soda or shake.
- Be aware that commercially prepared milkshakes often include sodium in their ingredients as well as whole milk and sugar.
- Ask for water if milk isn't available.

Dessert:

- Skip it! Or make it an occasional treat. Many of the dessert items are high in calories, fat, and sugar.
- Choose fresh fruit from the salad bar, if available, as an alternative.

ASK YOURSELF...

- Do I exercise regularly?
- What exercise could I add to my activities?
- Have I tried several diets that don't succeed in keeping lost pounds off?
- What common sense practices could I follow to control my weight?
- Do I know the ingredients in my favorite snacks?
- What are my favorite desserts—the ones I eat most frequently?
- How can I change desserts to reduce calories and add nutrients?
- What foods can I eat at snack and dessert times to add nutrients I need to my diet?
- What kinds of restaurants do I eat in? How can I choose healthier foods from the menu?
- Are there other restaurants I can try that allow better choices?

Try these recipes for desserts and snacks—

Pumpkin Cupcakes

Try these cupcakes unfrosted for a nutrient-plus dessert. The pumpkin is high in vitamin A and the raisins add iron.

24 cupcakes

Per cupcake:

Calories	140
Total fat	5 grams
Saturated fatty acids	1 gram
Cholesterol	27 milligrams
Sodium	130 milligrams

Whole-wheat flour	1-1/2 cups
All-purpose flour	1 cup
Sugar	3/4 cup
Baking powder	2 tablespoons
Ground cinnamon	2 teaspoons
Ground nutmeg	1/2 teaspoon
Salt	1/4 teaspoon
Eggs, slightly beaten	3
Skim milk	1 cup
Vegetable oil	1/2 cup
Canned pumpkin	1 cup
Raisins, chopped	3/4 cup
Vanilla	1 tablespooon

1. Preheat oven to 350°F.
2. Place 24 paper baking cups in muffin tins.
3. Mix dry ingredients thoroughly.
4. Mix remaining ingredients; add to dry ingredients. Stir until dry ingredients are barely moistened.
5. Fill paper cups two-thirds full.
6. Bake about 20 minutes or until toothpick inserted in center comes out clean.
7. Remove from muffin tins and cool on rack.
8. Freeze cupcakes that will not be eaten in the next few days.

Oatmeal Applesauce Cookies

Applesauce adds moistness to this low-calorie, lowfat, and low-sodium version of oatmeal cookies.

About 5 dozen cookies

Per cookie:

Calories	45
Total fat	2 grams
Saturated fatty acids	Trace
Cholesterol	0
Sodium	35 milligrams

All-purpose flour	1 cup
Baking powder	1 teaspoon
Ground allspice	1 teaspoon
Salt	1/4 teaspoon
Margarine	1/2 cup
Sugar	1/2 cup
Egg whites	2
Rolled oats, quick-cooking	2 cups
Unsweetened applesauce	1 cup
Raisins, chopped	1/2 cup

1. Preheat oven to 375°F.
2. Grease baking sheet.
3. Mix flour, baking powder, allspice, and salt.
4. Beat margarine and sugar until creamy. Add egg whites; beat well.
5. Add dry ingredients.
6. Stir in oats, applesauce, and raisins. Mix well.
7. Drop by level tablespoonfuls onto baking sheet.
8. Bake 11 minutes or until edges are lightly browned.
9. Cool on rack.

Peanut Butter-Date Spread

The dates and juice make this peanut butter-date spread lower in fat and calories per tablespoon than plain peanut butter. However, it is still fairly high in fat, so balance it out with lower fat choices elsewhere.

About 3/4 cup

Per tablespoon:

Calories	80
Total fat	5 grams
Saturated fatty acids	1 gram
Cholesterol	0
Sodium	Trace

"No-salt-added" peanut butter	1/2 cup
Dates, chopped	1/3 cup
Orange juice	3 tablespoons
Orange rind, grated	1/4 teaspoon

1. Mix all ingredients.
2. Use as a spread on melba toast or lowfat crackers.

Food Facts for Older Adults

Questions Older People Ask

5

New information about nutrition seems to come out each day. Often, the information does not address the concerns of older adults. This section answers some common questions older people ask about nutrition.

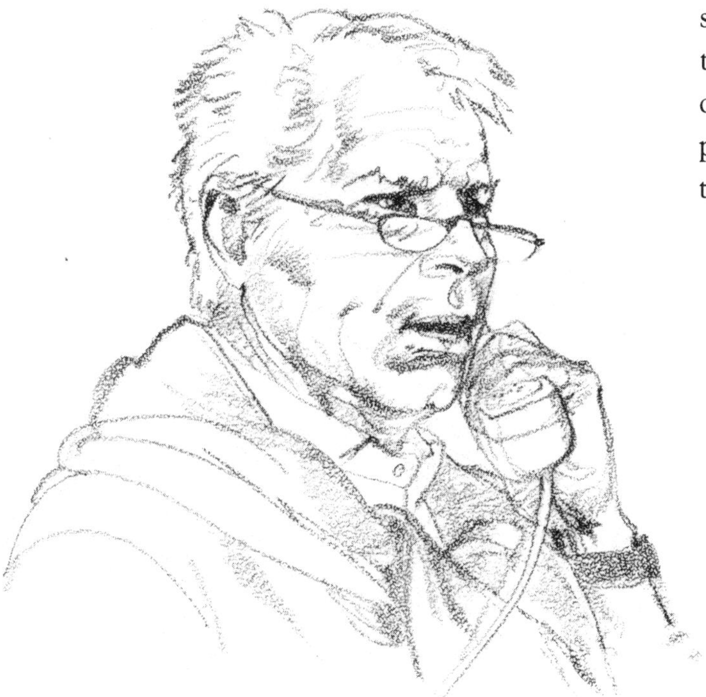

Are there any foods or vitamins that can help prevent memory loss?

As of now, there is no reliable evidence that any foods or vitamins can help prevent memory loss such as occurs in Alzheimer's disease. Choline and lecithin have been tried to treat Alzheimer's, but neither was successful. People with Alzheimer's are at a greater risk for developing nutritional deficiencies, which can cause additional problems. Other kinds of severe memory loss and confusion are caused by excessive alcohol intake or by a deficiency of vitamin B-12 or folate. A B-12 deficiency can sometimes be reversed by injections of this vitamin. It's important for anyone showing signs of memory loss and confusion to have a complete checkup, including a nutritional evaluation. Ask your health care provider.

Is there such a thing as "good cholesterol"?

You may have heard the terms "good cholesterol" and "bad cholesterol." These terms refer to substances called lipoproteins, which are "transport vehicles" that carry cholesterol in the blood. There are several kinds of lipoproteins. High-density lipoprotein (HDL) is often called the "good" kind because it removes cholesterol from the bloodstream, carrying it to the liver. The "bad" kind of cholesterol is transported by low-density lipoprotein (LDL). This is the cholesterol that gets deposited inside the arteries, where it may build up over time and eventually block the flow of blood. High levels of LDL increase your risk of heart disease, while high HDL levels lower your risk.

Diet can affect levels of LDL and HDL in the blood, but there are no foods that contain these substances. A cholesterol screening usually tells you the **total** amount of cholesterol circulating in your blood, but not how much of it comes from HDL and LDL. If your total cholesterol level is over 200 mg/dl and you have other risk factors for heart disease, your doctor may request another blood test to find out what your HDL and LDL levels are. This test must be done after you fast for 12 hours. Talk with your doctor about how the various components of blood cholesterol affect your risk.

ABC
Health Clinic
Blood Cholesterol Report

Name: Jane Doe	Date Drawn: 10/1/92		Date Rec'd: 10/1/92
Sex: F Age: 66	Date of Report: 10/3/92		
Test Name	Result	Units	Reference Range
Cholesterol	222	mg/dl	149—229
HDL Cholesterol	72	mg/dl	30—80
LDL Cholesterol	140	mg/dl	60—178

I have trouble with my teeth and gums and have difficulty eating raw vegetables. How can I get enough fiber?

Cooked vegetables and fruits also supply fiber in your diet, as do cooked cereals and baked goods that contain whole grains. These will be much easier to chew. See your dentist or ask for a referral to one who specializes in dental problems of older adults. Much can be done to help your teeth and gums to make eating a variety of foods more enjoyable.

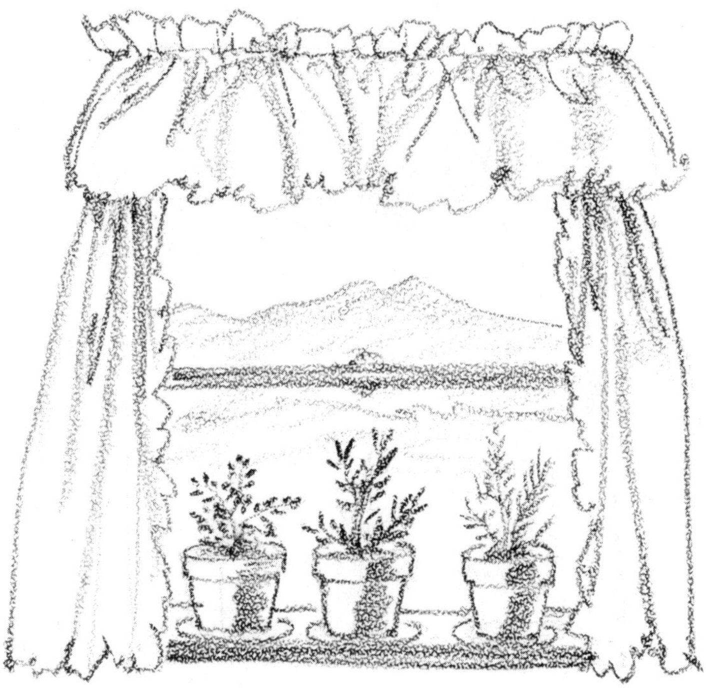

Things just don't taste good to me, so I have no interest in eating. What can I do to perk up my appetite?

People often find that their senses of taste and smell get duller as they age. As a result, they may overload their food with salt or even lose interest in food. Be creative with herbs, spices, and lemon juice. They all add flavor that can perk up your taste again. Experiment with different spices to see what appeals to you. You may even want to try growing fresh herbs, either in your garden or in a pot on a sunny windowsill. Trying new recipes and choosing colorful foods in a variety of textures may also add interest to your meals.

I hate eating alone and as a result, I often skip meals. How can I make eating interesting?

Eating alone can be boring and sometimes even depressing. Many people don't want to spend time preparing meals just for themselves. Make an effort to make meals enjoyable. Try some of these ideas:

- Plan meals, set the table, light candles, play music, or eat when a television show you like is on. You deserve the same effort and care in preparing your own meals as the guests you might serve for a dinner party.

- Invite friends over for meals. You could each bring a part of the meal or trade portions of "planned leftovers."

- Eat out once a week or so. Many restaurants have lower prices and smaller portions at lunchtime. Some may offer reduced prices for older adults. Plan a daytime outing with a friend — go to lunch and visit a museum or attend an afternoon concert or theater performance. (See Section 4 for hints on making healthy food choices when you eat out.)

- Visit a senior center at lunchtime; participate in meals offered through your local agency on aging.

- Form a gourmet club with others who eat alone.

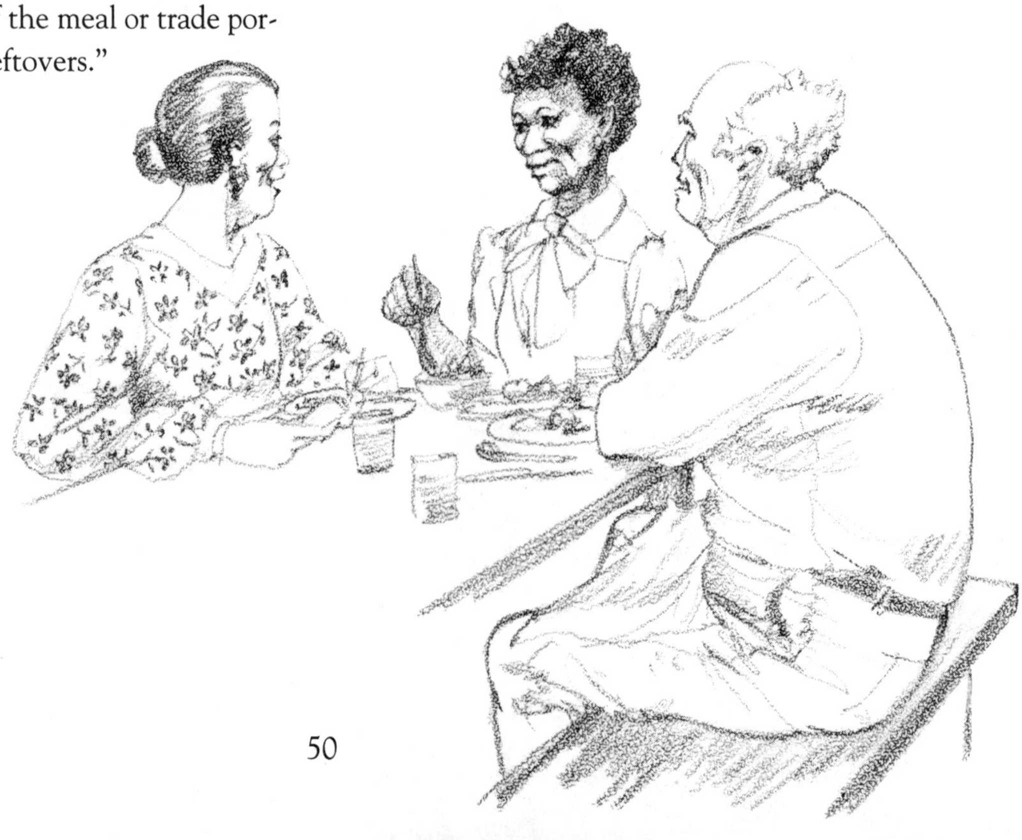

I've never liked eating breakfast. Do I need to eat breakfast to have a healthy diet?

It's not necessary to eat a big meal first thing in the morning. The important goal is to eat a balanced diet that includes foods from all the food groups each day. Set an eating pattern that works for you. For example, perhaps you like a mid-morning snack instead of a formal breakfast. Just be sure to make it a healthy snack, such as fruit and a muffin or toast. Often, people who skip meals eat too many snacks filled with empty calories.

What can I eat to help my arthritis?

Unfortunately, there is no food that relieves the pain of arthritis, but scientists are doing a lot of research in this area. You may see advertisements for food products or supplements that promise relief, but in truth they won't help you. A balanced diet will contribute to your overall good health, and avoiding too much weight will put less strain on your joints. There are also many simple tools such as jar openers that you can use to help you with everyday tasks. Contact your local chapter of the Arthritis Foundation, listed in the telephone book, for more information.

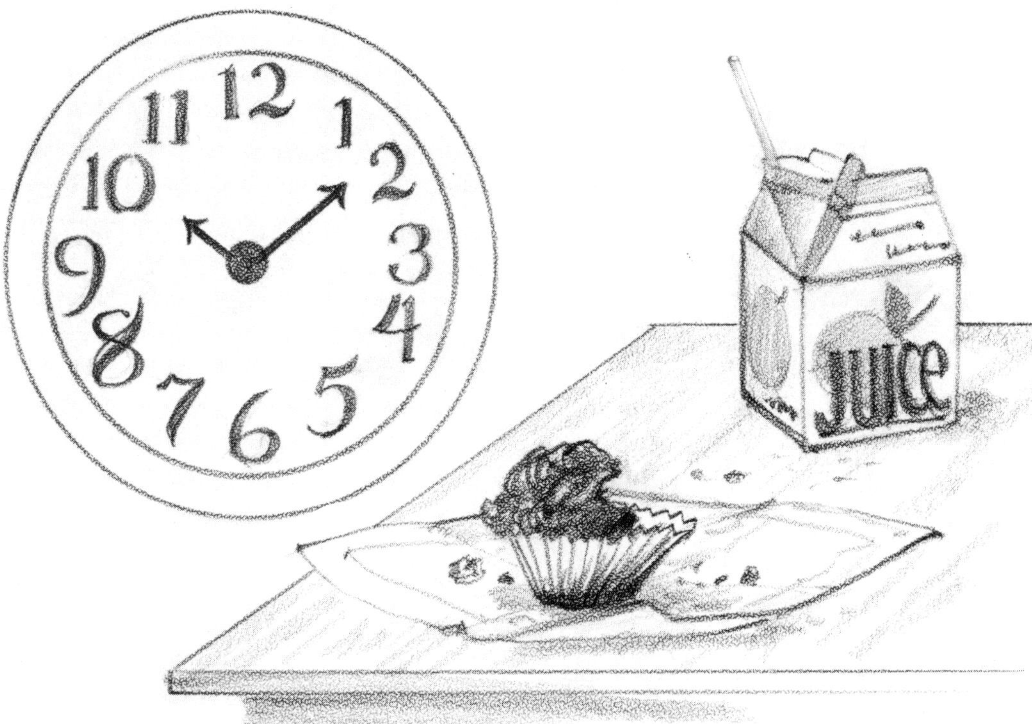

Can I always believe what I read in the newspaper?

New research about diet and health often gets in the newspaper or appears on the evening news, but no matter how promising or discouraging this news may be, making changes in your diet based on a single report is not wise. Government agencies and health organizations, such as the U.S. Departments of Agriculture and of Health and Human Services (USDA and DHHS), the National Academy of Sciences, and the American Heart Association, base their recommendations on dozens of studies carried out over many years. These groups continuously review new research findings and make recommendations only when there is widespread agreement among experts. Consult the resource list included in this bulletin for sources of more information.

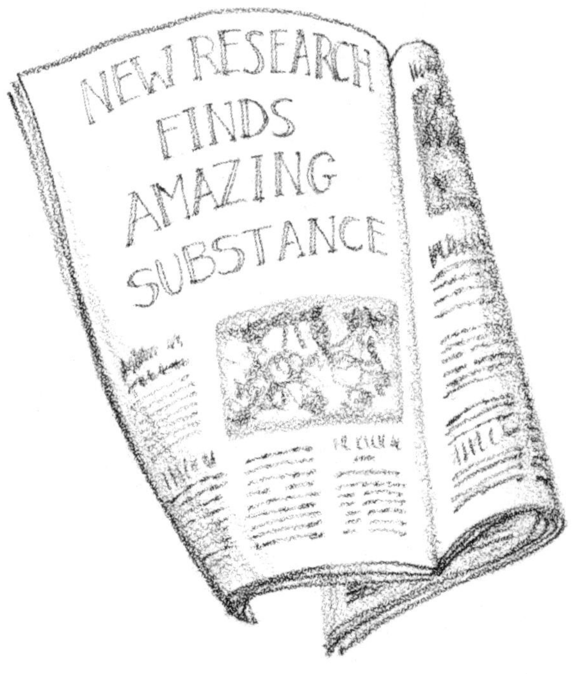

How do I know when a claim that a food product or supplement cures diseases is true?

These claims can be dangerous because they often prevent users from getting the medical help they need. They also create false hopes and waste money. In general, if it sounds too good to be true, it is. Suspect a product if it—

- makes outrageous claims, like curing a disease or reversing the aging process. No product or food has yet been proven to do either.
- promises immediate or fast results.
- does not list ingredients.
- cites only one study or a preliminary study as proof of results.
- does not give information about possible side effects.
- claims to be a secret formula.
- is available only from one source.

I don't eat many dairy products. How can I get enough calcium?

People who have trouble digesting milk can usually drink it in small amounts or can drink milk to which the enzyme lactase has been added (see Section 2 for suggestions). Buttermilk, yogurt, or cheese are good alternatives and are easier to digest. Other people simply don't like milk or dairy products. Calcium can be found in other foods. It's found naturally in leafy green vegetables like kale and broccoli. It's also added to some products such as fruit juice. It's best to get as much calcium as you can from the food you eat. If you feel you are not getting enough from foods, discuss whether you should take a calcium supplement (and what kind) with your doctor or dietitian.

> ***DID YOU KNOW???***
>
> One baked potato (even without the skin) has 610 mg of potassium; one banana (well-known as a good source of potassium) has 450 mg.

I take diuretics; how can I get enough potassium?

First of all it's important to know if the diuretic you take is one that depletes potassium or one that has little effect on it. Generally, the more potent diuretics produce significant potassium losses. You should discuss the specific drug you are taking with the doctor who prescribed it for you. Most people's diets do not provide enough potassium to make up for what is lost due to the diuretic. However, proper choice of foods can effectively replace potassium losses.

Most foods provide some potassium. Fruits, vegetables, milk, and yogurt are among the best sources. Some meats, poultry, and fish are good sources too. Here are some common foods that are good sources of potassium:

- bran cereals
- cooked dried fruit such as apricots, peaches, prunes
- bananas
- potatoes, baked or boiled
- sweetpotatoes, pumpkin, winter squash
- stewed tomatoes
- lima beans
- cooked dry beans, peas, lentils
- milk and yogurt (all types)

Any Other Questions ...

Write your own questions below. Check the resource list in section 7 for people who may be able to answer your questions.

Food Facts for Older Adults

Tips and Recipes

6

You don't have to eliminate all of the fat, sugar, and sodium from the foods you eat to follow a healthy diet. Balance is the key. Think about how you can cut down on the fat, sugar, and sodium in the foods you prepare and eat. Consider also how you can get more whole grains, fruits, and vegetables. Simple changes make a difference. The following pages contain tips on preparing foods with less fat, sugar, and sodium as well as recipes to help you eat in a more healthful way.

Some Ideas for Better Eating

Make some simple changes in your recipes, using the recipes in this section as examples.

Notice that—

- Many of the recipes are prepared without added salt. Some use ingredients that already contain salt such as canned tuna, cereal, cheese, and soy sauce, while others are seasoned with herbs or spices.
- Lower fat ingredients are used instead of similar ingredients that are higher in fat. For example, water-packed tuna instead of oil-packed tuna, reduced-calorie salad dressing instead of regular salad dressing, skim milk instead of whole milk, and chicken breast without skin rather than chicken breast with skin.
- The desserts and quick bread are prepared with less sugar than most similar recipes.
- Whole-grain products are used in place of some or all of the all-purpose flour.

Make some simple changes at the table, too. See if you can take the salt shaker away or cut down the number of times you use it. Do you usually add a dab of butter or margarine to vegetables when you put them on the table? Try a low-calorie spread instead. Are there other changes you can make?

Tips About Breads, Cereals, Rice, and Pasta...

- Choose products made with whole grains often; for example, whole-wheat, oatmeal, oat-bran, pumpernickel, and rye breads, and cornmeal products, such as corn tortillas.
- Cook pasta and rice without salt or fats. Try using unsalted broth or tomato juice to add flavor.
- Try flavored pastas now available at many grocery stores, such as whole-wheat, spinach, or herb pasta.
- Try brown rice; it has more flavor and more fiber.
- Make a pasta salad for dinner or lunch. It's easy to make and puts leftovers to good use. Just go easy on the mayonnaise or use reduced-calorie mayonnaise or salad dressing.

Tuna Pasta Salad

This salad is a tasty change from a typical tuna salad. It provides a serving of cooked pasta and half a serving of fruit in addition to the tuna.

4 servings, about 1 cup each

Per serving:

Calories 195
Total fat .... 2 grams
Saturated fatty acids .... Trace
Cholesterol .... 13 milligrams
Sodium .... 170 milligrams

Elbow macaroni, uncooked	3/4 cup
Tuna, water-pack, drained	6-1/2-ounce can
Celery, thinly sliced	1/2 cup
Seedless red grapes, halved	1 cup
Salad dressing, mayonnaise-type, reduced-calorie	3 tablespoons

1. Cook macaroni according to package directions, omitting salt. Drain.
2. Toss macaroni, tuna, celery, and grapes together.
3. Mix in salad dressing.
4. Serve warm or chill until served.

Menu Suggestion: Serve with broccoli spears, pumpernickel rolls, and ice milk topped with sliced strawberries.

Bran Apple Bars

Apples and bran cereal add dietary fiber. Using egg whites in place of a whole egg keeps cholesterol to a trace.

16 bars

Per bar:

Calories..........110
Total fat..........4 grams
Saturated fatty acids..........1 gram
Cholesterol..........Trace
Sodium..........110 milligrams

Whole-bran cereal (see Note)	1 cup
Skim milk	1/2 cup
Flour	1 cup
Baking powder	1 teaspoon
Ground cinnamon	1/2 teaspoon
Ground nutmeg	1/4 teaspoon
Margarine	1/3 cup
Brown sugar, packed	1/2 cup
Egg whites	2
Apple, pared, chopped	1 cup

1. Preheat oven to 350 °F.
2. Grease 9- by 9-inch baking pan.
3. Soak bran in milk until milk is absorbed.
4. Mix dry ingredients thoroughly.
5. Beat margarine and sugar until creamy. Add egg whites; beat well. Stir in apples and bran mixture. Add dry ingredients; mix well.
6. Pour into pan.
7. Bake 30 minutes or until a toothpick inserted in center comes out clean.
8. Cool on rack.
9. Cut into 16 bars.

Note: Check the nutrition label of cereals for sodium content. Some whole-bran cereals contain almost twice as much sodium as others.

Zucchini Bread

This quick bread contains less fat, cholesterol, sugar, and sodium than many traditional squash breads. Use for dessert in place of an iced cake.

1 loaf, 18 slices, about 1/2-inch thick

Per slice:

Calories..........110
Total fat..........4 grams
Saturated fatty acids..........1 gram
Cholesterol..........0
Sodium..........90 milligrams

Whole-wheat flour	1 cup
All-purpose flour	1 cup
Baking powder	1-1/2 teaspoons
Ground cinnamon	1 teaspoon
Baking soda	1/4 teaspoon
Salt	1/4 teaspoon
Egg whites	3
Sugar	1/2 cup
Vegetable oil	1/3 cup
Vanilla	1-1/2 teaspoons
Zucchini squash, coarsely shredded, lightly packed	2 cups

1. Preheat oven to 350 °F.
2. Grease 9- by 5- by 3-inch loaf pan.
3. Mix dry ingredients, except sugar.
4. Beat egg whites until frothy. Add sugar, oil, and vanilla. Continue beating for 3 minutes.
5. Stir in zucchini; mix lightly.
6. Add dry ingredients. Mix just until dry ingredients are moistened.
7. Pour into loaf pan.
8. Bake 40 minutes or until toothpick inserted in center comes out clean.
9. Cool on rack. Remove from pan after 10 minutes.
10. To serve, cut into 18 slices about 1/2-inch thick.

Tips About Vegetables...

- Both raw vegetables and cooked vegetables provide dietary fiber. The less they are cooked, the more vitamins remain in the vegetables. Try steaming them just to the point that they are tender but crisp.

- Eat potatoes with their skins for more fiber.

- Season vegetables with herbs, yogurt, and lemon juice. Limit butter, margarine, heavy dressing, honey, salt, and soy sauce.

- Canned vegetables are often high in sodium. Try some of the special low-sodium or "no-salt-added" versions.

- Add beans, split peas, and lentils to your diet; they're an inexpensive source of protein and fiber. Add them to soups, stews, salads, and rice dishes.

Herbed Vegetable Combo

These steamed vegetables with herb seasonings add color and flavor to a meal without adding fat or salt.

4 servings, about 3/4 cup each

Per serving:

Calories..........25
Total fat..........Trace
Saturated fatty acids..........Trace
Cholesterol..........0
Sodium..........10 milligrams

Water	2 tablespoons
Zucchini squash, thinly sliced	1 cup
Yellow squash, thinly sliced	1-1/4 cups
Green pepper, cut into 2-inch strips	1/2 cup
Celery, cut into 2-inch strips	1/4 cup
Onion, chopped	1/4 cup
Caraway seed	1/2 teaspoon
Garlic powder	1/8 teaspoon
Tomato, cut into 8 wedges	1 medium

1. Heat water in large frypan.
2. Add squash, green pepper, celery, and onion.
3. Cover and cook over moderate heat until vegetables are tender-crisp—about 4 minutes.
4. Sprinkle seasonings over vegetables. Top with tomato wedges. Cover and cook over low heat until tomato wedges are just heated—about 2 minutes.

Tips About Fruits...

- Fruits offer natural sweetness with the added benefits of fiber, vitamins, and minerals.
- Use fresh or canned fruit slices as a colorful garnish for main dishes, salads, and cereals.
- Blend fresh, plain frozen, or canned fruit with milk for a fruitshake.
- Add dried fruit to muffins and quick breads.
- Eat fresh fruits topped with yogurt and sprinkled with cinnamon.
- Bake or broil apples, pears, or bananas with cinnamon and nutmeg; fruit tastes even sweeter when eaten while warm.

Apple Crisp

Whole-wheat flour and rolled oats add dietary fiber. Using less sugar and fat than in an old-fashioned apple crisp recipe means lower sugar and fat content per serving.

4 servings, 1/2 cup each

Per serving:

Calories..........235
Total fat..........9 grams
Saturated fatty acids..........2 grams
Cholesterol..........0
Sodium..........105 milligrams

Tart apples, pared, sliced	4 cups
Water	1/4 cup
Lemon juice	1 tablespoon
Brown sugar, packed	1/4 cup
Whole-wheat flour	1/4 cup
Old-fashioned rolled oats	1/4 cup
Ground cinnamon	1/2 teaspoon
Ground nutmeg	1/4 teaspoon
Margarine	3 tablespoons

1. Place apples in 8- by 8- by 2-inch baking pan.
2. Mix water and lemon juice, pour over apples.
3. Mix sugar, flour, oats, and spices.
4. Add margarine to dry mixture; mix until crumbly.
5. Sprinkle crumbly mixture evenly over apples.
6. Bake at 350 °F until apples are tender and topping is lightly browned, about 40 minutes.

Tips About Milk, Yogurt, and Cheese...

These foods are an important source of calcium but can add fat and extra sodium to your diet.

- Choose lower fat and lower sodium versions often, such as:
  - * skim milk
  - * evaporated skim milk
  - * lowfat or nonfat plain yogurt
  - * whipped cottage cheese for dips and dressings
  - * part skim ricotta or mozzarella
  - * lowfat process cheeses
  - * lower sodium cheeses

- If you don't like to drink milk, try using it in soups and puddings (see the following recipe for broccoli soup).

Broccoli Soup

This recipe has less sodium and fat than canned broccoli soup. Using unsalted broth and adding 1/4 teaspoon salt results in less sodium than using a salted broth and no salt.

4 servings, about 1 cup each

Per serving:

Calories............110

Total fat............3 grams

Saturated fatty acids............2 grams

Cholesterol............9 milligrams

Sodium............250 milligrams

Broccoli, chopped (see Note)	1-1/2 cups
Celery, diced	1/4 cup
Onion, chopped	1/4 cup
Chicken broth, unsalted	1 cup
Skim milk	2 cups
Cornstarch	2 tablespoons
Salt	1/4 teaspoon
Pepper	Dash
Ground thyme	Dash
Swiss cheese, shredded	1/4 cup

1. Place vegetables and broth in saucepan. Bring to boiling, reduce heat, cover, and cook until vegetables are tender—about 8 minutes.
2. Mix milk, cornstarch, salt, pepper, and thyme; add to cooked vegetables. Cook, stirring constantly, until soup is slightly thickened and mixture just begins to boil.
3. Remove from heat. Add cheese and stir until melted.

Note: A 10-ounce package of frozen chopped broccoli can be used in place of fresh broccoli. The soup will have about 120 calories and 260 milligrams of sodium per serving.

Tips About Meat, Poultry, and Fish...

- You don't have to eliminate red meat, or any one meat, from your diet. Lean, trimmed beef is low in fat and supplies important amounts of minerals such as iron and zinc.

- Choose leaner types of meat:
  * beef—round, loin, sirloin, and chuck arm steaks or roasts, especially "select" grade cuts (often labeled in supermarkets as "lean")
  * pork—tenderloin, center loin roasts and chops
  * veal—roasts and chops
  * lamb—leg, loin roasts and chops, and foreshanks
  * chicken and turkey, especially light meat
  * most fish; choose tuna canned in water when available
  * shellfish

- Try substituting ground turkey or chicken for ground beef in casseroles and other dishes.

- Try dishes made with dry beans and peas as occasional alternatives. Dry beans and peas are low in fat and provide protein and minerals similar to lean meat, poultry, and fish. They also provide dietary fiber.

- Limit your use of processed meats such as hotdogs, sausage, and luncheon meats. They are usually high in both sodium and fat. Choose more lowfat or lower salt versions.

- Keep the fat and sodium content low when you prepare meats:
  * trim visible fat and remove the skin from poultry
  * broil and bake instead of fry
  * place meat on a rack when cooking so fat can drain away from the meat
  * cook with no added fat in nonstick pans
  * baste meats with unsalted broth, tomato juice, or fruit juice instead of fatty drippings, or marinate before cooking
  * cool stews and soups before serving so you can skim fat off the top
  * limit sauces and gravies that are high in saturated fats, such as cream sauce
  * use onion or garlic powder instead of seasoned salts
  * season with herbs and spices
  * use commercially prepared sauces sparingly; they are usually high in sugar or sodium or both

- Modify recipes so you use smaller amounts and leaner cuts of meat and more of other ingredients like potatoes, rice, noodles, grains, or vegetables.

Beef & Vegetable Stirfry

Using a lean meat cut, round steak, and only 1 teaspoon of oil keeps the fat lower than in a traditional stirfry.

4 servings, about 3/4 cup each

Per serving:

Calories..........145
Total fat..........4 grams
Saturated fatty acids..........1 gram
Cholesterol..........44 milligrams
Sodium..........300 milligrams

Beef round steak, boneless	3/4 pound (12 ounces)
Vegetable oil	1 teaspoon
Carrots, sliced	1/2 cup
Celery, sliced	1/2 cup
Onion, sliced	1/2 cup
Soy sauce	1 tablespoon
Garlic powder	1/8 teaspoon
Pepper	Dash
Zucchini squash, cut in thin strips	2 cups
Cornstarch	1 tablespoon
Water	1/4 cup

1. Trim all fat from steak. Slice steak across the grain into thin strips about 1/8-inch wide and 3 inches long. (Partially frozen meat is easier to slice.)
2. Heat oil in frypan. Add beef strips and stirfry over high heat, turning pieces constantly, until beef is no longer red—about 3 to 5 minutes. Reduce heat.
3. Add carrots, celery, onion, and seasonings. Cover and cook until carrots are slightly tender—3 to 4 minutes.
4. Add squash; cook until vegetables are tender-crisp—3 to 4 minutes.
5. Mix cornstarch and water until smooth. Add slowly to beef mixture, stirring constantly.
6. Cook until thickened and vegetables are coated with a thin glaze.

Chicken & Vegetable Stirfry

VARIATION

Per serving:

Calories..........140
Total fat..........2 grams
Saturated fatty acids..........Trace
Cholesterol..........51 milligrams
Sodium..........320 milligrams

Use 3 chicken breast halves without bone or skin (about 12 ounces of raw chicken) in place of beef. Slice into thin strips. Chicken should be cooked until thoroughly done or no longer pink in color.

Chicken Italiano

This colorful chicken main dish is quick and easy to prepare. All ingredients are cooked together in a single pan.

4 servings, 1 chicken breast half and 3/4 cup of spaghetti mixture each

Per serving:

Calories.....280
Total fat.....3 grams
Saturated fatty acids.....1 gram
Cholesterol.....68 milligrams
Sodium.....320 milligrams

Chicken breast halves, skinned, boned	4
Vegetable oil	1 teaspoon
Thin spaghetti, broken into fourths	4 ounces (about 1-1/2 cups dry)
Onion, cut in wedges	1 small
Green pepper, cut in strips	1 small
Instant minced garlic	1/8 teaspoon
Oregano leaves	1 teaspoon
Salt	1/8 teaspoon
Pepper	1/8 teaspoon
Bay leaf	1
Tomatoes	16-ounce can
Water	1/4 cup
Parsley, chopped	1 tablespoon, if desired

1. Pound chicken breasts with a metal mallet between sheets of plastic wrap until about 1/2-inch thick.
2. Heat oil in frypan. Brown chicken breasts on each side.
3. Add spaghetti, onion, and pepper strips around chicken. Sprinkle with seasonings.
4. Break up large pieces of tomatoes. Pour tomatoes and water over top of chicken.
5. Bring to boiling. Reduce heat, cover, and cook until chicken and spaghetti are done, about 15 minutes.
6. Remove bay leaf. Garnish with parsley.

Menu Suggestion: Serve with spinach-mandarin orange salad with reduced-calorie dressing and garlic bread (small amount of soft margarine and garlic powder).

Turkey Italiano

VARIATION

Per serving:

Calories.....275
Total fat.....3 grams
Saturated fatty acids.....Trace
Cholesterol.....70 milligrams
Sodium.....305 milligrams

Use 1 pound raw turkey breast fillets or tenderloins in place of chicken. (Bone and skin are already removed.)

Broiled Sesame Fish

For a quick, lowfat main dish, try this fish recipe. It takes about 15 minutes to prepare and contains very little fat.

4 servings, about 2-1/2 ounces each

Per serving:
Calories..........110
Total fat..........3 grams
Saturated fatty acids..........Trace
Cholesterol..........46 milligrams
Sodium..........155 milligrams

Cod fillets, fresh or frozen	1 pound
Margarine, melted	1 teaspoon
Lemon juice	1 tablespoon
Dried tarragon leaves	1 teaspoon
Salt	1/8 teaspoon
Pepper	Dash
Sesame seed	1 tablespoon
Parsley, chopped	1 tablespoon

1. Thaw frozen fish in refrigerator overnight or defrost briefly in a microwave oven. Cut fish into four portions.
2. Place fish on a broiler pan lined with aluminum foil. Brush margarine over fish.
3. Mix lemon juice, tarragon leaves, salt, and pepper. Pour over fish.
4. Sprinkle sesame seeds evenly over fish.
5. Broil until fish flakes easily when tested with a fork—about 12 minutes.
6. Garnish each serving with parsley.

Dilled Fish Fillets

Using dill weed and lemon juice for flavor in place of butter or margarine keeps the fat low.

4 servings, about 2-1/2 ounces each

Per serving:
Calories..........90
Total fat..........1 gram
Saturated fatty acids..........Trace
Cholesterol..........45 milligrams
Sodium..........130 milligrams

Frozen haddock or cod fillets	1 pound
Lemon juice	1 tablespoon
Dried dill weed	1/8 teaspoon
Salt	1/8 teaspoon
Pepper	Dash

1. Thaw frozen fish in refrigerator overnight or thaw in microwave oven. Separate into four fillets or pieces.
2. Place fish in heated frypan. Sprinkle with lemon juice and seasonings.
3. Cover and cook over moderate heat until fish flakes when tested with a fork, about 5 minutes.

Menu Suggestion: Serve with braised carrots and celery, new potatoes boiled in skin, and applesauce muffins made from mix.

MICROWAVE INSTRUCTIONS: Place fish in a glass baking dish. Cover with wax paper. Cook at "medium" power for 3 minutes. Remove cover, turn fish over, and sprinkle with lemon juice and seasonings. Cover and continue cooking at "medium" power for 3 minutes or until fish flakes with a fork.

Modifying Your Recipes

Here's an example of how to use these tips. The recipe below shows simple adjustments in a typical beef stroganoff recipe that can help you moderate fat and cholesterol.

Changes from typical recipe:

- Use a less fatty meat cut—round steak in place of sirloin—and trim fat from meat.
- Use buttermilk in place of sour cream.
- Use a nonstick pan and no butter to cook the meat.
- Prepare gravy with buttermilk instead of butter.

Light Beef Stroganoff

4 servings, 1/2 cup of stroganoff and 1/2 cup of noodles each

Per serving:

Calories	275
Total fat	6 grams
Saturated fatty acids	2 grams
Cholesterol	71 milligrams
Sodium	325 milligrams

Beef round steak, boneless, trimmed	3/4 pound
Fresh mushrooms	1/4 pound
Onion, sliced	1/2 cup
Beef broth, condensed	1/2 cup
Water	1/2 cup
Catsup	1 tablespoon
Pepper	1/8 teaspoon
Flour	2 tablespoons
Buttermilk	1 cup
Noodles, cooked, unsalted	2 cups (about 2-1/2 cups uncooked)

1. Slice steak across the grain into thin strips, about 1/8-inch wide and 3 inches long. (It is easier to cut thin slices of meat if it is partially frozen.)
2. Wash and slice mushrooms.
3. Cook beef strips, mushrooms, and onion in **nonstick** frypan until beef is lightly browned.
4. Add broth, water, catsup, and pepper. Cover and simmer until beef is tender, about 45 minutes.
5. Mix flour with about 1/4 cup of the **buttermilk** until smooth; add remaining buttermilk. Stir into beef mixture. Cook, stirring constantly, until thickened.
6. Serve over noodles.

For each serving, these changes result in savings of 240 calories, 24 grams total fat, 15 grams saturated fatty acids, and 62 milligrams cholesterol.

Adapt Your Staples for Better Health...

You can reduce fat and sodium in the boxed products you use, such as macaroni and cheese. Just follow the chart below:

Mix	Changes	Serving size (cup)	Fat saved per serving (grams)	Sodium saved per serving (milligrams)
Macaroni and cheese	● *Omit salt when cooking macaroni.* ● *Use lowfat milk.* ● *Reduce added margarine by half.*	3/4	6	265
Seasoned rice and rice/pasta mixtures	● *Reduce added margarine by half.*	1/2	2	20
Bread stuffing	● *Reduce added margarine by half.*	1/2	4	45
Scalloped and au gratin potatoes	● *Use lowfat milk.* ● *Reduce added margarine by half.*	1/2	2	20

Note: Savings for macaroni and cheese and potatoes are for products made with 2 percent fat milk in place of whole milk. Reduce fat even further by using 1 percent fat or skim milk.

Food Facts for Older Adults

Want More Information???

7

For assistance in answering your questions about nutrition and health, contact the following organizations. If they cannot answer your questions directly, they will refer you to someone who can.

Administration on Aging
330 Independence Avenue, S.W.
Washington, DC 20201
(202) 619-0724

U.S. Government agency that provides information on health and aging programs, offered through State and area agencies on aging.

Alzheimer's Association
Suite 1000
919 N. Michigan Avenue
Chicago, IL 60611
(312) 335-8700
1(800) 272-3900 toll-free hotline

Offers a hotline that provides information and assistance for families coping with Alzheimer's disease.

American Association of Retired Persons
1909 K Street, N.W.
Washington, DC 20049
(202) 434-2277

Membership organization for people over age 50, offering publications and volunteer-run programs on a variety of economic, social, and health issues.

American Dietetic Association
Suite 800
216 West Jackson Boulevard
Chicago, IL 60606
(312) 899-0040

Professional organization offering assistance in locating a registered dietitian in your community.

American Geriatrics Society
Suite 300
770 Lexington Avenue
New York, NY 10021
(212) 308-1414

Professional organization of physicians with geriatric training, offering assistance in locating a doctor in your community with special training in treating older adults.

Arthritis Foundation
1314 Spring Street, N.W.
Atlanta, GA 30309
(404) 872-7100

Provides information and programs on arthritis, including treatment options and self-help materials for those with arthritis and their families.

Food and Drug Administration
Office of Consumer Affairs
5600 Fishers Lane, HFE 88
Rockville, MD 20857
(301) 443-3170

U.S. Government agency that answers questions about the safety of food additives, drugs, and medical devices.

Human Nutrition Information Service
USDA
6505 Belcrest Road
Hyattsville, MD 20782
(301) 436-5724

U.S. Government agency that provides information on using the Dietary Guidelines and preparing foods.

National Institute on Aging
Public Information Office
Federal Building, Room 6C12
9000 Rockville Pike
Bethesda, MD 20892
(301) 496-1752

U.S. Government agency that provides information on health and other issues of interest to older people.

National Cancer Institute
Office of Cancer Communications
Building 31, Room 10A24
9000 Rockville Pike
Bethesda, MD 20892
1(800)422-6237 toll-free hotline

U.S. Government agency that provides information on cancer prevention and treatment.

National Heart, Lung, and Blood Institute
Information Office
Building 31, Room 4A21
9000 Rockville Pike
Bethesda, MD 20892
(301) 496-4236

U.S. Government agency that conducts research and provides information about heart, lung, and blood diseases.

Office of Disease Prevention and Health Promotion
National Health Information Center
P.O. Box 1133
Washington, DC 20013-1133
1(800) 336-4797

U.S. Government agency that operates a clearinghouse and hotline to provide health information and referrals.

☆ U.S. GOVERNMENT PRINTING OFFICE: 1993 348-309/80193